Elizabeth Connor, MLS, AHIP

Internet Guide to Travel Health

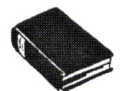

*Pre-publication
REVIEWS,
COMMENTARIES,
EVALUATIONS...*

"This comprehensive Internet source guide to travel health is the first on the topic. It contains descriptive evaluations of more than 400 high-quality Web sites on travel health. The selected Web sites are current and reliable, ranging from general travel health, to pre-travel planning, to specific issues and concerns on health when traveling, and travel diseases, conditions, and ailments. Sections which list sites on interactive travel tools, organizations, full-text publications, and other sources add value to the book. This book is an invaluable reference tool, highly recommended to all libraries. It is useful to anyone who is concerned about travel safety. Health care providers who advise patients on how to stay healthy during travel will find it very helpful."

Jie Li, MLS, AHIP
*Medical Center Site Coordinator,
Biomedical Library,
University of South Alabama*

"Do library patrons need information on vaccines needed before traveling to Zaire? Do they need help in dealing with travel anxiety? What do you need to know to ship your dog across the state, the country, or to Great Britain? What will the weather be like tomorrow in the region to which you are traveling? For any of these and thousands more questions that come up in planning or recovering from a trip, Connor's book provides an excellent and easy-to-use source on where to go on the World Wide Web to get your answers. It is an essential addition to the reference collection of any library serving patrons who have or will travel, and is a good buy for any individual or groups who travel frequently."

Michael R. Kronenfeld, MLS, MBA, AHIP
*Director, Learning Resource Center,
A. T. Still University of the Health Sciences*

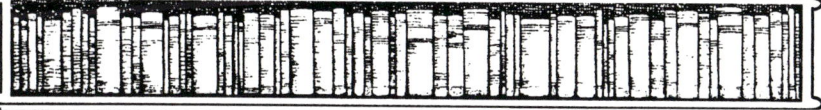

More pre-publication
REVIEWS, COMMENTARIES, EVALUATIONS . . .

"The savvy traveler who consults the Web before embarking on his or her journey will find it an easier task using Elizabeth Connor's *Internet Guide to Travel Health*. This annotated guide of carefully researched health-related Web sites reviews for every traveler—from the globe-trotter to the armchair variety—essential information on traveling in good health. Professionals who advise the traveler also will find it useful. Of the sites listed, those which the author considers 'authoritative and original in content' are indicated by a representational graphic.

Internet Guide to Travel Health not only lists sites for pretravel information, for those traveling with children or pets, and for those traveling with preexisting medical problems, it also details sites for those who go abroad seeking medical treatment or recuperation. Real-time sites are given; worldwide organizations—many publishing travel alerts—are listed, as are sites which publish full-text, health-related documents. This book is a thoughtful compendium of information not only on how to remain healthy as you travel, but also how to travel health aware. As you plan your trip and whether or not your laptop travels with you, *Internet Guide to Travel Health* is for you!"

Sally Brown, MLIS
*Reference Librarian,
Health Sciences Library,
West Virginia University,
Morgantown*

"Question: 'Why buy a book containing travel health Web sites when I can search the Internet myself?' Answer: Connor, experienced medical librarian and international traveler, has produced the most comprehensive volume of authoritative Web sites for travel health. Whether you are planning your first cruise, a cross-country auto trip, or an international tour, Connor recommends sites to answer your questions about diseases, such as allergies and asthma, malaria, SARS, hepatitis, diarrhea, and West Nile virus, and the health issues of required immunizations and vaccinations, foodborne illnesses, jet lag, exercise and fitness, and travel with children, disabilities, and pets.

Internet Guide to Travel Health contains sites for general travel health, pretravel planning, as well as interactive tools for last-minute questions on weather, safety, and travel alerts. Full-text sites lead the travel planner to guides, reports, and newsletters. In the Introduction, Connor provides an overview of searching the Internet, including anatomy of Web site addresses and evaluation of Web sites. A useful glossary is included.

This book is recommended for public library reference collections, travel agencies, public health departments, and especially for frequent and adventure travelers."

Janet S. Fisher, MLS, AHIP
*Medical Librarian, James H. Quillen College of Medicine Library,
Johnson City, Tennessee*

More pre-publication
REVIEWS, COMMENTARIES, EVALUATIONS . . .

"*Internet Guide to Travel Health* is an excellent resource of Internet sites providing the consumer with an impressive array of health information relating to travel. Whether you travel for work, pleasure, or adventure, this basic, easy-to-use, well-organized comprehensive sourcebook is a guide to a wealth of wellness information, as well as to information on specific health issues, concerns, and conditions, and how to maintain good health away from home.

This book is a useful, handy compilation of links providing the potential to improve health knowledge and health risks, whether traveling near or far. It is a valuable resource to consult for pretravel planning. Do you want to stay healthy on a cruise? Calculate jet lag and learn how to manage it at your new destination? Do you know what to pack in your travel medicine kit? This book provides sources for advice and answers to these and many more questions, from preparing for medical emergencies on the road or abroad, to taking medications, medical devices, and paraphernalia through customs. This book is strongly recommended for those who travel, for those who dream of travel, and for all concerned with good health."

Anne K. Robichaux, MSLS, AHIP
Professor Emerita and Former Associate Director of Libraries, Medical University of South Carolina

"This publication is a comprehensive guide to essential Internet resources for anyone planning a trip, concerned about traveling, or curious about health and safety conditions around the globe. The guide starts with an informative and extensive introduction discussing helpful information on Web site addresses, what to do if a site address is not working, how to evaluate health Web sites, and searching on the Web.

This book includes a very unique section on interactive tools, with essential travel planning sites from AAA, AccuWeather, and the CDC. This section also includes an online health records secure site, run by WebMD and accessible from anywhere, for travelers to enter their health history, allergies, immunizations, and other information.

Internet Guide to Travel Health is a well-organized resource with many sites that will be essential references for any traveler. Now that I have read this guide, I will not plan a trip or travel abroad without consulting it first for my health, safety, and peace of mind."

Amelia Butros, MLS, AHIP
*Chair, International Cooperation Section, Medical Library Association;
Assistant Director, Scripps Institution of Oceanography Library*

The Haworth Information Press®
An Imprint of The Haworth Press, Inc.
New York • London • Oxford

NOTES FOR PROFESSIONAL LIBRARIANS
AND LIBRARY USERS

This is an original book title published by The Haworth Information Press®, an imprint of The Haworth Press, Inc. Unless otherwise noted in specific chapters with attribution, materials in this book have not been previously published elsewhere in any format or language.

CONSERVATION AND PRESERVATION NOTES

All books published by The Haworth Press, Inc. and its imprints are printed on certified pH neutral, acid free book grade paper. This paper meets the minimum requirements of American National Standard for Information Sciences-Permanence of Paper for Printed Material, ANSI Z39.48-1984.

Internet Guide to Travel Health

THE HAWORTH INFORMATION PRESS
Internet Guides to Consumer Health Care
M. Sandra Wood, MLS
Editor

The Guide to Complementary and Alternative Medicine on the Internet by Lillian R. Brazin

Internet Guide to Travel Health by Elizabeth Connor

Internet Guide
to Travel Health

Elizabeth Connor, MLS, AHIP

The Haworth Information Press®
An Imprint of The Haworth Press, Inc.
New York • London • Oxford

Published by

The Haworth Information Press®, an imprint of The Haworth Press, Inc., 10 Alice Street, Binghamton, NY 13904-1580.

© 2004 by The Haworth Press, Inc. All rights reserved. No part of this work may be reproduced or utilized in any form or by any means, electronic or mechanical, including photocopying, microfilm, and recording, or by any information storage and retrieval system, without permission in writing from the publisher. Printed in the United States of America.

PUBLISHER'S NOTE
Due to the ever-changing nature of the Internet, Web site names and addresses, though verified to the best of the publisher's ability, should not be accepted as accurate without independent verification.

Cover design by Lora Wiggins.

Library of Congress Cataloging-in-Publication Data

Connor, Elizabeth, MLS.
    Internet guide to travel health / Elizabeth Connor.
        p. ; cm.
    Includes bibliographical references and index.
    ISBN 0-7890-1597-8 (hard : alk. paper) — ISBN 0-7890-1824-1 (soft : alk. paper)
    1. Travel—Health aspects—Computer network resources.
    [DNLM: 1. Travel—Resource Guides. 2. Communicable Disease Control—Resource Guides. 3. Information Services—Resource Guides. 4. Internet—Resource Guides. 5. Safety—Resource Guides. QT 29 C752i 2004] I. Title.
RA783.5.C665 2004
025.06'61368—dc22
                                                                                                    2004012031

To the talented library staff
of the Ross University School of Medicine
in Portsmouth, Dominica

Thank you for working with me
to create a productive and supportive workplace,
and for teaching me so much about your hopes and dreams.

Bless you.

ABOUT THE AUTHOR

Elizabeth Connor, MLS, AHIP, holds an adjunct faculty position in the Daniel Library at The Citadel in Charleston, South Carolina. She has held library leadership positions at major teaching hospitals and academic medical centers in the United States and abroad, and is a distinguished member of the Academy of Health Information Professionals. Ms. Connor spent more than eight years living and working as a medical library director in two developing countries: the Commonwealth of Dominica and the Kingdom of Saudi Arabia.

Ms. Connor has authored several peer-reviewed articles about medical informatics, electronic resources, search engines, and chat reference, and has written more than fifty book reviews for *Library Journal, Against the Grain, Journal of the Medical Library Association, Medical Reference Services Quarterly,* and *The Post and Courier.* Over the past ten years, she has delivered more than eighteen paper and poster presentations at international and national library conferences. She has served as the Associate Editor (International) for the *Bulletin of the Medical Library Association,* and currently manages the book review process for *Medical Reference Services Quarterly.*

CONTENTS

Chapter 1. Introduction — 1
Anatomy of a Web Site Address — 1
Evaluating Web Content — 3
Using Search Engines/Directories — 4
Staying Healthy and Well — 6

Chapter 2. General Travel Health Sites — 7

Chapter 3. Pretravel Planning — 23
Checklists — 23
Health Certificates and Other Documents — 25
Immunizations and Vaccinations — 27
Medications, Devices, and Supplies — 31
Predeparture Health Examinations — 32
Travel Health Insurance — 32

Chapter 4. Specific Issues and Concerns — 35
Accidents — 35
Automobile Travel — 36
Bus or Train Travel — 39
Children Traveling Alone and Traveling with Children — 40
Contraindications to Travel — 42
Cruise Ship Travel — 44
Death — 45
Disabilities — 45
Evacuation Services — 48
Health Tourism — 49
Medical Care While Traveling — 50
Medications — 51
Natural Disasters — 52
Pets Traveling Alone and Traveling with Pets — 53
Quarantine — 59
Seniors Traveling Alone and Traveling with Seniors — 60
Weather — 62
Women Traveling Alone — 63

Chapter 5. Diseases, Conditions, and Ailments   65

   Air Rage and Road Rage   65
   Allergies and Asthma   66
   Altitude Sickness   68
   Arthritis   68
   Back Problems   69
   Bites and Stings   70
   Cold Weather Conditions   71
   Deep Vein Thrombosis   72
   Dengue Fever and Other Hemorrhagic Fevers   75
   Dental Problems   75
   Diabetes   76
   Diarrhea   77
   Ear Problems   78
   Exercise Before and During Travel   79
   Fear of Flying   80
   Food-Borne Illnesses   81
   Hepatitis   82
   HIV and AIDS   83
   Jet Lag   84
   Lung Diseases   85
   Lyme Disease   88
   Mad Cow Disease   89
   Malaria   89
   Motion Sickness   90
   Pregnancy   91
   Sunburn, Sunstroke, and Heat Exhaustion   93
   West Nile Virus   95
   Yellow Fever   96

Chapter 6. Interactive Tools   99

Chapter 7. Organizations   107

Chapter 8. Full-Text Publications   115

Glossary   135

Suggested Readings   143

Index   145

A man travels the world over in search of what he needs and returns home to find it.

George Moore (1852-1933)

Chapter 1

Introduction

People travel the world for a variety of reasons, including pleasure, business, work, and education. The ease of traveling thousands of miles in less than a day's time exposes us to myriad health risks caused by different organisms, populations, flora and fauna, food and drink, time zones, and climate changes. Healthy and safe travel involves planning, preparation, and the awareness of situations and potential health risks.

Vacationers, business travelers, explorers, and health care professionals alike seek authoritative, reliable, and up-to-date information to stay well and to prevent a variety of diseases and ailments while traveling in the United States and abroad. Discerning individuals use the Internet to find updated and authoritative information on a variety of topics. This compilation of Web sites serves as a handy, useful, and easy-to-consult guide for persons traveling near or far, or for armchair travelers. The emphasis is on English-language travel information for North Americans, with some links from Australia, the United Kingdom, and other European countries.

ANATOMY OF A WEB SITE ADDRESS

Hypertext transfer protocol (http) is the set of standards used to represent content on the World Wide Web. Although many Web browsers no longer require the http:// prefix when entering site addresses, other prefixes are understood by browser software to connect to other types of Internet resources. For example, the telnet:// prefix is used to establish a telnet connection, which allows remote log-ins to resources such as electronic catalogs. The ftp://

prefix uses file transfer protocol to transmit files from one computer to another. The gopher:// prefix is used to connect to gopher content, an Internet protocol and organizational structure that was developed before the World Wide Web. Each Web site address is comprised of distinct and meaningful parts that describe the host computer, directory, and file name:

<protocol://host.domain.suffix.suffix/directory>

For example, in the address <http://healthlink.mcw.edu/travel-medicine/>, the host name is Healthlink; the domain is Medical College of Wisconsin (MCW), which is an educational institution (.edu); and the directory is travel-medicine. In the address for MedlinePlus's Traveler's Health section, <http://www.nlm.nih.gov/medlineplus/travelershealth.html>, the domain is the National Library of Medicine (NLM) at the National Institutes of Health (NIH), a group of government agencies (.gov); the directory is MedlinePlus; and the file name is travelershealth.

Web site addresses use a variety of organizational and geographic suffixes that are meaningful. Table 1.1 lists common Web site address suffixes and their meanings. The ease with which Web sites are designed and content can be uploaded has resulted in many temporary, redesigned, or outdated sites. Dead links result when a site changes file names, alters the site navigation, or stops publishing. If a particular site address no longer functions, delete the /directory, /filename.htm, or /filename.html part of the address, and use just the host.domain.suffix parts. After the site

TABLE 1.1. Site Type and Geographic Suffixes

Site Type Suffix	Geographic Suffix
.com—Commercial sites	.au—Australia
.edu—Educational sites	.ca—Canada
.gov—Government sites	.ch—Switzerland
.mil—Military sites	.ie—Ireland
.net—Commercial sites that provide network services	.uk—United Kingdom
.org—Organization or association sites	.us—United States

loads, use the site's search function to find the specific document or section needed.

There is nothing inherently suspicious or problematic about medical content featured on commercial Web sites or sites with a .com suffix at the end of the address. Reputable educational institutions such as the Mayo Clinic and The Johns Hopkins University, for example, maintain authoritative consumer health information on .com sites with content that is separate from their .edu sites. Some excellent consumer health sites sell brochures and other publications, but the sites featured in this guide provide freely available information, including some sites that require completion of a registration process to personalize future site interactions.

EVALUATING WEB CONTENT

Consumers of health information should be particular and skeptical about medical information or advice obtained through the Internet. The currency, accuracy, and source of health-related information are very important factors to consider. Laypersons should be as discerning as health professionals when distinguishing between anecdotal information and content derived from authoritative and peer-reviewed sources.

Health on the Net (HON) Foundation (http://www.hon.ch/) is an organization based in Switzerland that developed MedHunt, an English/French medical search engine, and a set of standards for evaluating sites with medical content. The HON Code of Conduct rates Web sites according to whether a particular site with medical content

- explains qualifications for dispensing advice or developing content;
- maintains confidentiality when handling medical information;
- attributes information derived from other sources;
- indicates the date content was modified or revised;
- lists contact information for content developers;

- identifies sources of funding or sponsorship;
- explains the use of advertisements or sale of products; and/or
- distinguishes original informational content from promotional content.

USING SEARCH ENGINES/DIRECTORIES

Although Internet applications were developed originally to allow government agencies to communicate and share information with one another and date back to 1969, the World Wide Web was not introduced until 1990. Gopher, the first Internet search tool, appeared in 1991, but the development of graphical browser tools (Mosaic, Netscape) and search engines/directories accelerated the growth, development, and acceptance of the World Wide Web.

The proliferation of search engines/directories has helped the Web evolve into a tool for daily living, but, too often, a typical search query yields thousands of marginally relevant results with many dated or extinct links. Search engines have advantages and drawbacks, and it is worthwhile to learn the features of a few to serve a variety of needs.

A search engine delivers dynamically generated results based on the words typed into the search box. Search directories are somewhat static groupings of categorized sites and tend to be smaller in scope than search engines. For subjects related to travel health, it may be more productive to focus on several sites with reliable health content (Centers for Disease Control and Prevention, National Library of Medicine's MedlinePlus, University of Maryland Medicine, World Health Organization) than to enter keywords into search engine interfaces and spend hours sorting through links of dubious quality or authority.

Search engines/directories vary greatly in size and in how they are compiled, updated, and organized. Search Engine Showdown (http://www.searchengineshowdown.com/) and Search Engine Watch (http://searchenginewatch.com/) are excellent sources of information about how specific search tools work and the relative size, advantages, and features of each. The following search engines/directories are useful for searching a variety of topics and were used to locate links described in this book:

- **Google** (http://www.google.com/): Google is an excellent all-purpose resource for searching or browsing content, including publicly accessible Web sites, news group messages, images, and news information. The subject categories in the Google Directory (http://directory.google.com/) can be browsed and searched. Google's size is estimated at more than 2 billion pages; it includes caches of old pages and provides links to similar content.
- **All the Web** (http://www.alltheweb.com/): All the Web is considered one of the top search engines at 2.1 billion pages and is a close second to Google in terms of ease of use and comprehensiveness. Use this search engine if Google does not deliver the results expected.
- **Yahoo!** (http://www.yahoo.com/): Yahoo! is the first Web search directory and although it is small in size (approximately 2.5 million pages), its advantages include compilation by humans, organization, and ease of use. If Yahoo! exhausts its index, it refers the search query to another search engine. At the time of this writing, Yahoo!'s secondary search engine was Google.
- **Teoma** (http://www.teoma.com/): Although Teoma is smaller than other top-rated engines at 1 billion pages indexed, it proves its worth by delivering relevant results. Useful features include clustering results retrieved from the same site and additional hits accessible through a link to more results.

A number of specialized search engines and directories that focus on specific areas of interest, such as government or medicine:

- **FirstGov.gov** (http://www.firstgov.gov/): FirstGov is the U.S. government's Web portal, an aggregated interface to content on federal sites.
- **MedHunt** (http://www.hon.ch/medhunt/): Health on the Net Foundation (HON), also known for its approval system for health-related sites, developed this medical search engine.

- **SearchEdu.com** (http://searchedu.com), **SearchMil.com** (http://searchmil.com), **SearchGov.com** (http://searchgov.com): Despite the .com suffix on each of these sites, the interfaces retrieve results that are limited to .edu, .mil, and .gov sites, respectively.

The Invisible Web refers to content not easily accessed by normal search engines because of the way the information is organized and how search engines find links. To tease out valuable content featured in deeper layers of sites or within some Web-based databases, try Search Adobe PDF Online (http://searchpdf.adobe.com), InfoMine (http://infomine.ucr.edu/), Invisible Web (http://www.invisibleweb.com/), or Spire Project Light (http://spireproject.com/spir.htm).

STAYING HEALTHY AND WELL

Healthy People 2010 (http://www.healthypeople.gov/) is an effort organized by the Office of Disease Prevention and Health Promotion and other U.S. federal agencies to encourage American citizens to take personal responsibility for their health. Now more than at any other time in history, health knowledge, preventive measures, and treatments are available to improve and extend the quality of life for all.

The Internet has the potential to improve health knowledge and to increase awareness of health risks. Although this guide is intended to be as thorough as possible, use the sites marked with the ☑ symbol to save considerable time and effort when planning your travels. Consult the glossary to learn the definitions of words that are unfamiliar.

As a young girl growing up in New York, I dreamed of traveling the world and collecting souvenirs of my travels. I have had the good fortune to travel throughout the United States, Canada, and many countries, and to live overseas, without experiencing any travel-related diseases. I wish you healthy and safe journeys wherever your dreams take you.

Chapter 2

General Travel Health Sites

The sites included in this chapter cover many aspects of travel health, and are excellent resources for exploring various topics related to staying healthy while traveling. Consult the more specific chapters in this book to focus on individual issues, concerns, or medical conditions. The symbol ☑ is used to denote major resources with authoritative and original content.

Ask NOAH About: Travel and Vacations and Your Health
<http://www.noah-health.org/english/wellness/healthy living/travel.html>

New York Online Access to Health (NOAH) is a consumer health site developed by several New York–area university and public libraries that features authoritative content in English and Spanish. NOAH's travel section features links to other sites about trip planning, specific travel ailments, travel complications, traveling with pets, and more.

BluePrint for Health
<http://blueprint.bluecrossmn.com/topic/travelhealth>

BlueCross BlueShield of Minnesota hosts a consumer health site called BluePrint with information helpful to persons planning to travel. Sections include traveling with children, jet lag, economy class syndrome, and travelers with specific conditions. The site is well-designed, and it is easy to print and send content by e-mail.

British Airways Travel Clinics
<http://www.britishairways.com/travel/HEALTHCLIN INTRO/public/en_>

British Airways operates three travel clinics in the central London area and dispenses travel health advice to British Airways customers and noncustomers alike. This site features information about immunizations and staying well during flights.

☑ CDC Travelers' Health
<http://www.cdc.gov/travel/>

Developed and maintained by the National Center for Infectious Diseases, this site is accessible through the Centers for Disease Control and Prevention (CDC) site (see Figure 2.1). The Traveler's Health section provides authoritative information about destinations, outbreaks, diseases, vaccinations, safe food and water, traveling with children, traveling with pets, special needs travelers, cruise ships, and air travel. Reference materials include *Health Information for International Travel* (the "Yellow Book"), the "Blue Sheet," which summarizes health information for international travel, and the "Green Sheet," which summarizes sanitation inspections of cruise ships.

Combined Health Information Database (CHID)
<http://chid.nih.gov/>

CHID is a bibliographic database that combines the consumer health efforts of U.S. government agencies. Typical search results yield bibliographic citations to consumer health publications available from a variety of sources.

Dr. Mark Wise's The Travel Clinic
<http://www.drwisetravel.com/>

Dr. Mark Wise, a Canadian physician who trained at the London School of Tropical Medicine and Hygiene, operates a travel clinic in Thornhill, Ontario, Canada. This site offers practical advice about culture shock; jet lag; barefoot walking; personal

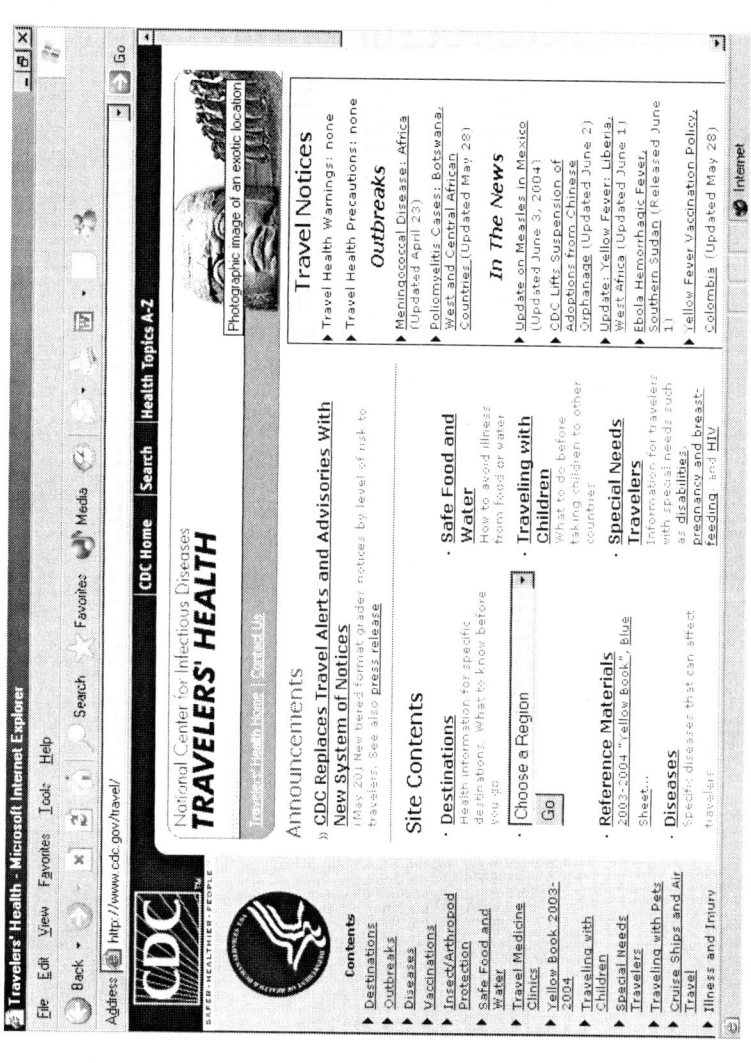

FIGURE 2.1. Travelers' Health, National Center for Infectious Diseases, U.S. Centers for Disease Control and Prevention Web Site

safety; motion sickness; diarrhea; tick-borne diseases; special-needs travelers with inflammatory bowel diseases, diabetes, pregnancy, or HIV/AIDS; and other topics.

☑ Fitfortravel
<http://www.fitfortravel.scot.nhs.uk/>

Developed by the Travel Medicine Division at the Scottish Centre for Infection and Environmental Health (SCIEH) (http://www.show.scot.nhs.uk/scieh/), Fitfortravel features TRAVAX (http://www.travax.scot.nhs.uk/InfoPage.htm), an interactive database of travel health information for health professionals; an A to Z index of diseases, countries, and topics; and a world map (see Figure 2.2).

Foreign and Commonwealth Office Travel
<http://www.fco.gov.uk/>

The Foreign and Commonwealth Office (FCO) is the United Kingdom's government office responsible for foreign affairs policy. The site features information related to traveling to specific countries, including political climate, local customs, safety and security, required vaccinations, and contacting British consulates.

Global Health.gov
<http://www.globalhealth.gov/>

This site was developed by the Office of Global Health Affairs, part of the U.S. Department of Health and Human Services. Site features include a Calendar of Events, Global Health Headlines, Statements and Speeches, Reports and Publications, Country Information, World Health Statistics, Fact Sheets, the Surgeon General's Page, and links to useful sites.

Health Advice for Travellers
<http://www.doh.gov.uk/traveladvice/>

The British Department of Health offers information about reciprocal health care arrangements, health updates, immunizations, taking medicine out of the United Kingdom, health advice for

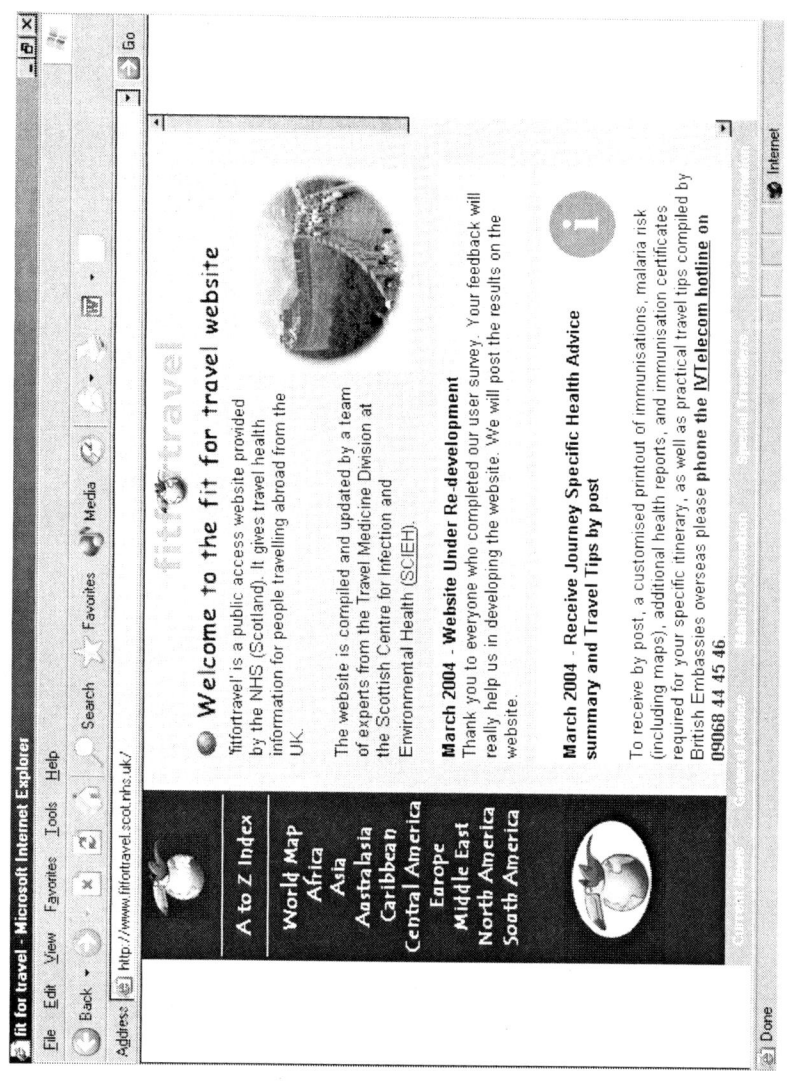

FIGURE 2.2. Fitfortravel, National Health Service (Scotland) Web Site

Muslim pilgrims, a country-by-country list of diseases, and other information specific to British citizens traveling abroad.

iJET Travel Intelligence
<http://www.ijet.com/index.html>

iJET describes itself as a travel risk management company, providing analysis of security risks around the world to travelers, expatriates, corporations, and other clients. The three types of travel alerts include critical alerts that will affect travel, warning alerts that may affect travel, and informational alerts, meaning that iJET is monitoring the situation. Typical security alerts include bombings in Israel and severe acute respiratory syndrome (SARS) outbreaks. Clients can order "itinerary-specific travel intelligence reports, real-time travel alerts and a personalized Web site" to be forwarded by e-mail or to a wireless device.

InteliHealth Healthy Travel to Distant Lands
<http://www.intelihealth.com/IH/ihtIH/WSIHW000/23722/20886/229189.html?d=dmtContent>

InteliHealth was developed by Aetna, the insurance company, and features Harvard Medical School's Consumer Health Information, including a channel called Healthy Travel to Distant Lands. Country-specific information features links to Centers for Disease Control and Prevention (CDC) information. Other information relates to pretrip vaccinations, avoiding mosquito-borne diseases, avoiding traveler's back, coping with traveler's diarrhea, and other topics.

International Medicine Center
<http://www.traveldoc.com/>

Edward Rensimer, MD, is the director of the International Medicine Center (IMC) in Houston, Texas. IMC promotes "awareness of international health and safety issues to corporate managers and medical departments." The IMC site features news and information about elderly travel, tuberculosis, bacterial meningitis, West Nile virus, severe acute respiratory syndrome (SARS), food and beverage safety, and health advisories delivered by e-mail. The site also sells region-specific travel medicine kits, including prescription and nonprescription medications and sterile supplies (syringes, suture materials, intravenous catheters, latex gloves) to prevent transmission of blood-borne pathogens.

Lonely Planet Health
<http://www.lonelyplanet.com/health/>

Lonely Planet is a site dedicated to exploration and travel. The health section of the Lonely Planet site includes information about predeparture planning (health insurance, medical kit, immunizations); keeping healthy (food and drink, water purification, nutrition); ailments related to heat, cold, altitude, or motion; specific infections and diseases; and cuts, bites, and stings.

☑ MASTA Online
<http://www.masta.org>

The London School of Hygiene and Tropical Medicine established Medical Advisory Services for Travellers Abroad (MASTA) in 1984. The MASTA site features useful information about immunizations, travel preparation, drugs to prevent diseases, travelers with special needs, and specific diseases associated with travel. Special features include a jet lag calculator. MASTA also sells an array of travel products, including insect repellents, mosquito netting, water purifiers, etc.

☑ MayoClinic.com
<http://www.mayoclinic.com/>

The renowned Mayo Clinic manages facilities in Rochester, Minnesota; Scottsdale, Arizona; and Jacksonville, Florida. Its excellent consumer health site does not have a special section devoted to travel health, but the search interface retrieves a number of topics of interest to travelers, and the Infectious Disease Center offers helpful advice for avoiding illness during travel.

MDtravelhealth.com
<http://www.mdtravelhealth.com/>

Intended for travelers and physicians alike, this site describes itself as "a limited liability corporation based in Scarsdale, N.Y.," with the content developed by David Goldberg, MD, a member of the International Society of Travel Medicine and the American Society of Tropical Medicine and Hygiene. Highlights include destination-specific health information summaries (recent outbreaks, medications, immunizations, food and water, insect protection, medical facilities, disaster preparedness, crime, traffic safety, embassy/consulate locations); information on infectious diseases from African trypanosomiasis to yellow fever; tips for illness prevention from altitude sickness to water purification; advice for special-needs travelers (infants and children, pregnant women, immunocompromised travelers, diabetics, and kidney patients); a list of travel health clinics by location; and health alerts sent by e-mail.

Medical College of Wisconsin HealthLink—Travel Medicine
<http://healthlink.mcw.edu/travel-medicine/>

HealthLink is the Medical College of Wisconsin's health promotion Web site. Health Link's Travel Medicine section includes detailed articles on a variety of topics, including a travel health risk overview, severe acute respiratory syndrome (SARS), scuba diving after blood clot, and others.

☑ MedlinePlus Traveler's Health
<http://www.nlm.nih.gov/medlineplus/travelershealth.html>

MedlinePlus is a consumer health information Web site developed and maintained by the U.S. National Library of Medicine (see Figure 2.3). The Traveler's Health section links to authoritative information related to health alert notices, vaccination certificate requirements, cruise ship travel, altitude illnesses, and MEDLINE results about travel health.

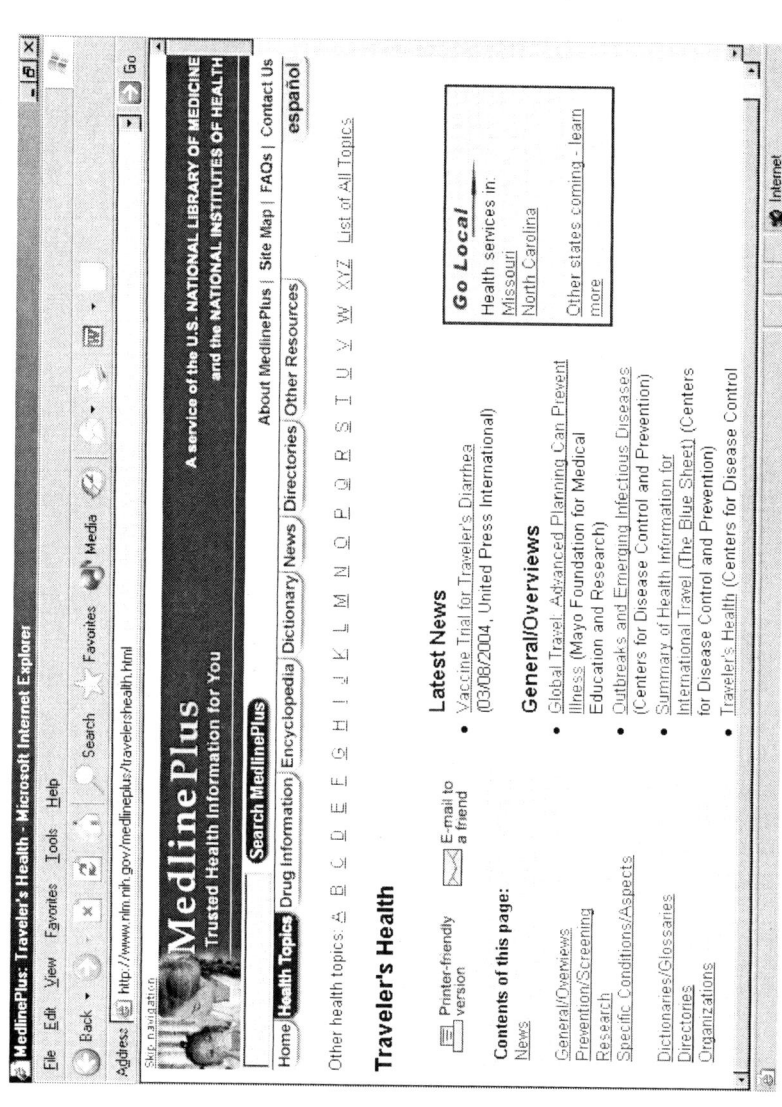

FIGURE 2.3. Traveler's Health, MedlinePlus Web Site

NetDoctor.co.uk
<http://www.netdoctor.co.uk/travel/index.shtml>

More than 250 physicians and health care professionals in the United Kingdom and Europe write the content included on the NetDoctor site. The site's Travel Medicine channel includes information about altitude sickness, crossing borders with medications, sun safety, malaria prevention, and other topics. Interactive features include discussion groups related to different subjects, online consultation with a doctor, and text messages sent by NetDoctor physicians to mobile telephones.

ProMED-mail
<http://www.promedmail.org/pls/askus/f?p=2400:1000>

ProMED-mail is the Program for Monitoring Emerging Diseases of the International Society for Infectious Diseases. Site features include Announcements, Recalls/Alerts, a Calendar of Events, Maps of Outbreaks, and Archives of Information. Announcements are listed in reverse chronological order. Outbreaks include West Nile virus, anthrax, influenza, and animal diseases.

TravDoc
<http://www.travdoc.com/>

TravDoc is a travel clinic located in Michigan. In addition to selling medical travel supplies, the clinic's site features information about traveling while pregnant (supplies, articles, research) and health and safety for expatriate workers. The site also contains articles discussing travel risks such as deep vein thrombosis, medical evacuation, traveler's diarrhea, and more.

The Travel Doctor
<http://www.thetraveldoctor.com/>

Developed and maintained by two physicians interested in travel medicine, this site includes travel tips and information about basic supplies, prescription medicines, crime, children, insects, sun exposure, malaria, food and water precautions, altitude, and water-related activities.

The Travel Doctor (TMVC)
<http://www.tmvc.com.au/>

The Travel Doctor (TMVC) is Australian-owned and operated. Travel Doctor staff include "specially trained doctors and nurses, specialist infectious diseases physicians, parasitologists, and public health physicians, all of whom have a keen interest in international health and travel medicine." The site includes health alerts; fact sheets; and information about travel security, deep vein thrombosis, severe acute respiratory syndrome (SARS), dengue fever, and other topics.

TravelHealth.co.uk
<http://www.travelhealth.co.uk/>

TravelHealth has partnered with the United Kingdom's Foreign and Commonwealth Office to provide information needed for British travelers to remain safe and healthy. Site features include pretravel advice; information about travel insurance, fear of flying, insect bites, sun safety, accident prevention, animal contact, disease prevention (malaria, dengue fever, cholera, tetanus, etc.), and vaccination requirements; and a list of travel clinics. The site also includes a pretravel questionnaire to be completed and taken to a local travel clinic.

TravelMedWeb
<http://www.travelmedicineweb.org/>

Intended for health care professionals, this site requires registration to access the content. Content includes feature articles on topics of interest to travelers (dengue fever, malaria treatment, the role of melatonin in jet lag); clinical case studies (rabies, hepatitis B, malaria); a journal club; and more.

University of Maryland Medicine—Travel Medicine
<http://www.umm.edu/travel/>

The University of Maryland Medicine site includes comprehensive travel medicine information. This site recommends that individuals anticipating foreign travel, especially to developing countries, establish a relationship with a travel medicine specialist rather than rely on the various travel alerts and other information available through U.S. government sites. That said, this site provides useful features, including immunization recommendations, U.S. State Department information, a traveler's guide, and information on common infectious diseases such as dengue fever, diarrhea, *E. coli* infection, hepatitis, yellow fever, etc.

☑ U.S. Department of State
<http://travel.state.gov/> and
<http://www.state.gov/travel/>

The U.S. Department of State maintains two sites of interest to travelers. The Bureau of Consular Affairs (http://travel.state.gov/) features headlines, travel warnings, public announcements, and consular information sheets (see Figure 2.4). Travel warnings are issued when the State Department determines that situations or conditions in a specific country pose a danger to U.S. citizens. Public announcements are more general in nature; for example, a typical public announcement cautions American citizens to be vigilant overseas. Consular information sheets feature a brief description of the country, entry/exit requirements, crime, medical facilities, the need for medical insurance, traffic safety and road conditions, an aviation safety oversight, customs regulations, criminal penalties, consular access, disaster preparedness, currency information, and other advice.

The U.S. Department of State's Travel and Living Abroad site (http://www.state.gov/travel/) includes some of the same links featured on the Bureau of Consular Affairs site (http://travel.state.gov/), as well as information about services for Americans abroad, dual citizenship, authentication of documents for use

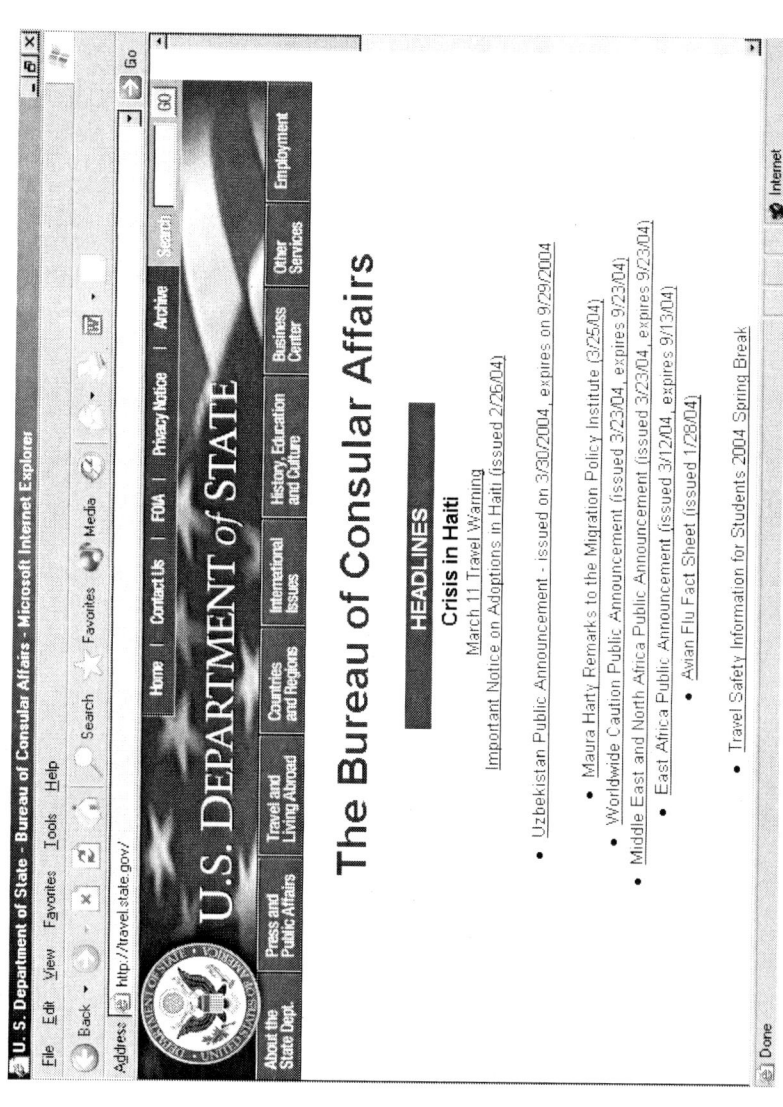

FIGURE 2.4. The Bureau of Consular Affairs, U.S. Department of State Web Site

abroad, and travel tips for students, women traveling alone, and older Americans (see Figure 2.5).

Well on the Road
<http://www.wellontheroad.com/index.html>

The Camino Medical Group International Travel Clinic in Sunnyvale, California, developed this site for "healthcare professionals and international travelers concerned with medical preparation for foreign travel." Site features include general information about travel-related illnesses (diarrhea, malaria, dengue fever, etc.); immunizations (hepatitis A, typhoid, yellow fever, etc.); medications (Cipro, Imodium, Malarone, etc.); and destinations (Afghanistan to Zimbabwe).

☑ World Health Organization (WHO)
<http://www.who.int/health_topics/travel/en/>

The World Health Organization (WHO) maintains a travel section within its site that features authoritative and up-to-date information about disease outbreaks; emergencies such as earthquakes, droughts, and other disasters in specific locations; vaccine-preventable diseases; health risks and precautions; and other information (see Figure 2.6).

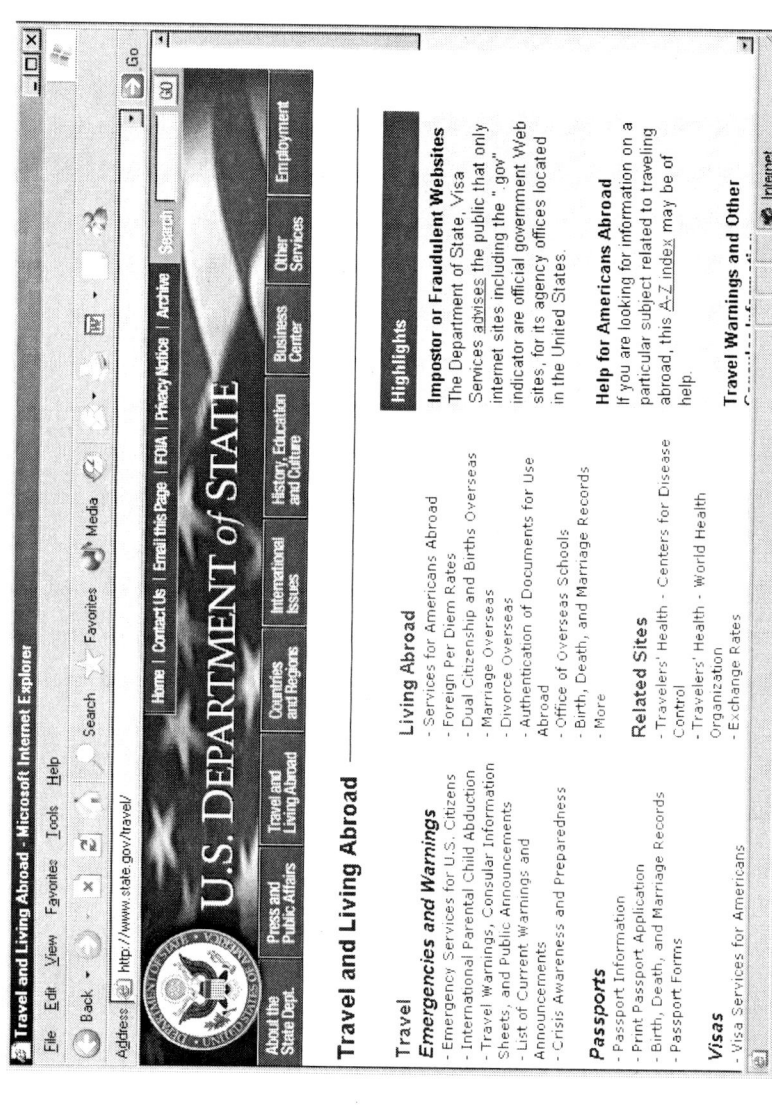

FIGURE 2.5. Travel and Living Abroad, U.S. Department of State Web Site

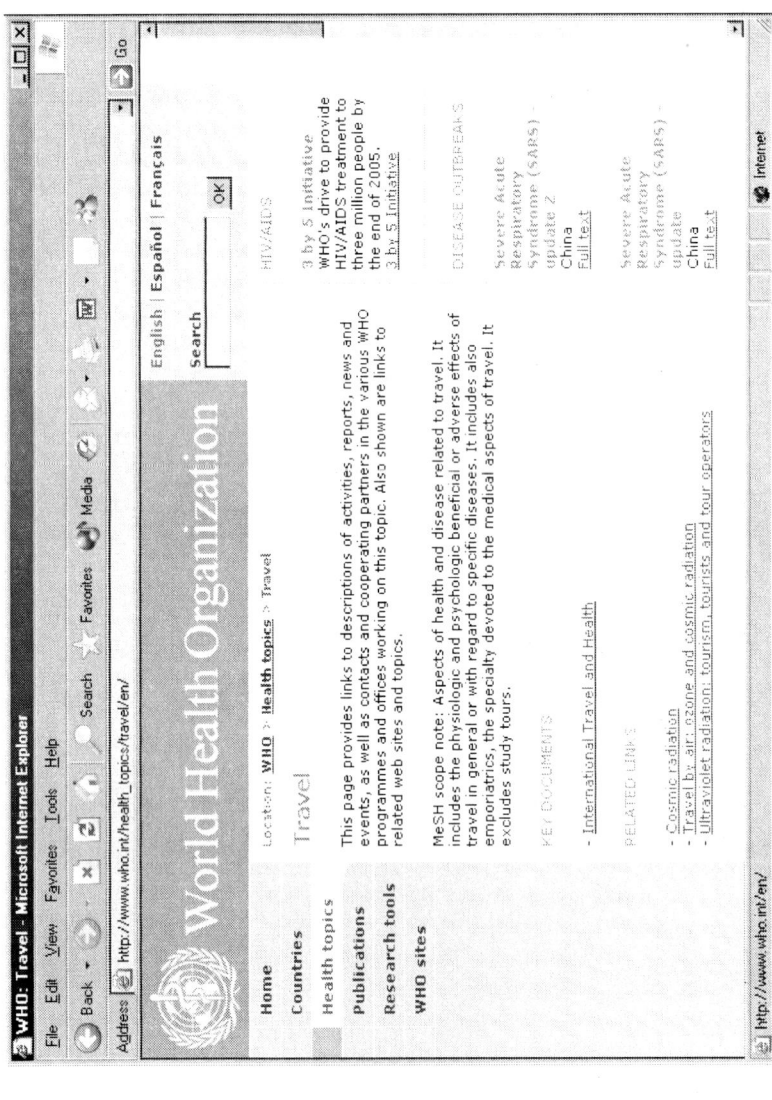

FIGURE 2.6. Travel, World Health Organization (WHO) Web Site

Chapter 3

Pretravel Planning

Regional and international travel can carry significant risk to personal health and safety. These links are useful for researching documentation, immunizations, and pretravel checkups required or recommended before humans and animals depart to specific locations. The symbol ☑ is used to denote major resources that feature authoritative and original content.

CHECKLISTS

☑ *Health Advice for Travellers*
<http://www.dh.gov.uk/PolicyAndGuidance/HealthAdviceToTravellers/fs/en>

The British Department of Health (DOH) developed this handy guide that covers world health risks, travel planning, and treatment while traveling (see Figure 3.1). The risk information explains the need for immunizations, food and drink precautions, outdoor safety, etc. The planning information discusses the need for checkups, first aid kits, insurance, etc. The treatment information covers Form E111, a document that allows citizens of European Economic Area (EEA) countries to seek emergency medical treatment in most European countries.

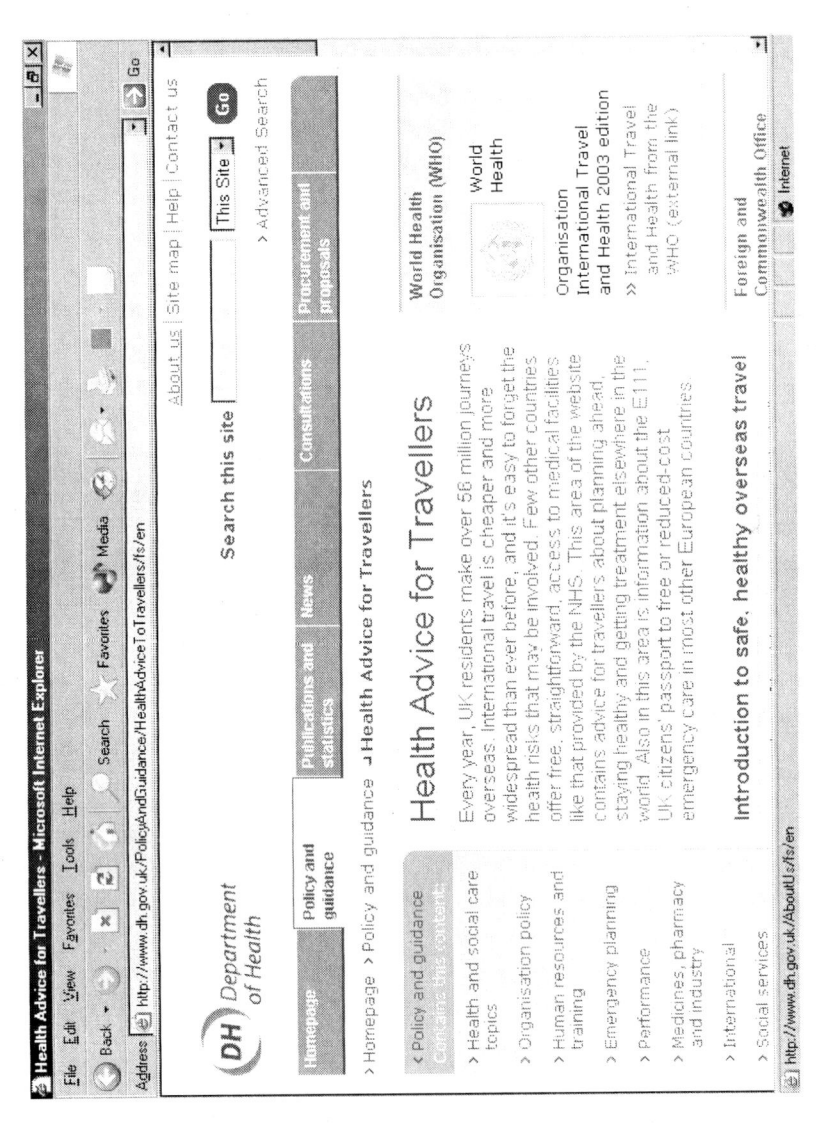

FIGURE 3.1. Health Advice for Travellers, British Department of Health Web Site

☑ International Checklist for the Traveller
<http://www.who.int/ith/chapter01_04.html>

Redesigned in 2002, this World Health Organization (WHO) resource provides useful information about the cause, transmission, geographical distribution, risk for travelers, prevention, and precautions for specific diseases from anthrax to yellow fever. The travel checklist suggests researching destination-specific risks and precautions and completing a predeparture medical questionnaire.

Pre-Departure Checklist
<http://www.umich.edu/~icenter/overseas/travel/checklist.html>

The International Center at the University of Michigan developed this predeparture checklist for traveling abroad. The checklist includes immunizations, travel advisories, and other items.

HEALTH CERTIFICATES AND OTHER DOCUMENTS

HIV Testing Requirements
<http://travel.state.gov/HIVtestingreqs.html>

The U.S. State Department explains that some countries require HIV test results for long-term visitors such as students or workers. The chart on this page lists countries alphabetically from Aruba to Yemen and their individual requirements for HIV testing.

International Certificate of Vaccination
<http://www.cdc.gov/travel/icv.htm>

The U.S. Centers for Disease Control and Prevention (CDC) site shows the front and back of the yellow International Certificate of Vaccination, also known as PHS-731, which is used to record dates of immunizations needed to travel to specific regions of the world. This document is approved by the World Health Organization and is published by the U.S. Public Health Service.

Passport for Healthy Travel
<http://wellness.ucdavis.edu/safety_info/on_the_move/passport_for_healthy_travel/>

The Wellness Center site of the University of California at Davis developed this simple page to help travelers plan healthy journeys. The checklist items suggest procedures to be done six months before departure as well as weeks and days ahead of time. There is a useful form for documenting names and contact information for home physician and pharmacist; medical conditions, allergies, and medications; and emergency contact information.

Traveling with HIV
<http://www.aegis.com/topics/travel.html>

AEGiS is the AIDS Education Global Information System. The information about traveling with HIV covers immunizations, HIV test results for travel to specific countries, and links to useful external sites.

☑ Vaccination Certificate Requirements
<http://www.cdc.gov/travel/vaccinations/cert-requirements2.htm>

This content about vaccination certificate requirements on the U.S. Centers for Disease Control and Prevention (CDC) site is derived from the CDC's *Health Information for International Travel 2003-2004*, better known as the "Yellow Book."

Vaccine Administration Record
<http://www.immunize.org/catg.d/p2023b.pdf>

The Immunization Action Coalition site provides a sample vaccine administration record to print and use for tracking the types and dates of specific immunizations.

IMMUNIZATIONS AND VACCINATIONS

☑ **Centers for Disease Control and Prevention: National Immunization Program**
   <http://www.cdc.gov/nip/>

Although the National Immunization Program section of the U.S. Centers for Disease Control and Prevention (CDC) site emphasizes routine child and adult immunization schedules, the site also includes information useful to world travelers, such as the quick reference vaccine chart (http://www.cdc.gov/nip/vaccine/vac-chart-public.htm), quick reference disease chart (http://www.cdc.gov/nip/diseases/disease-chart-public.htm), and vaccination certificate requirements (http://www.cdc.gov/travel/vaccinations/cert-requirements2.htm).

Guidelines for Vaccinating Pregnant Women
   <http://www.cdc.gov/nip/publications/preg_guide.htm>

Although the National Immunization Program section of the U.S. Centers for Disease Control and Prevention (CDC) emphasizes routine child and adult immunization schedules, the site also includes information useful to pregnant women planning to travel to areas that require additional immunizations. This fifteen-page guide was updated in October 2003.

Immunization Program
   <http://www.immunize-utah.org/public/pub_imm_travel.htm>

The Utah Department of Health Immunization Program site explains the need for immunizations for travel to specific regions of the world, provides a brief chart of specific immunizations, and includes links to useful external sites.

Immunization, Vaccines and Biologicals
<http://www.who.int/vaccines/>

The World Health Organization (WHO) information covers quality control on the use of biologicals for vaccine production, current research related to the subject, and a guide to travel vaccination.

Immunizations Recommended for Travel Outside of Canada
<http://www.hc-sc.gc.ca/pphb-dgspsp/tmp-pmv/236_e.html>

HealthCanada recommends specific immunizations for persons traveling outside of Canada.

National Network for Immunization Information (NNii)
<http://www.immunizationinfo.org/>

NNii, based in Alexandria, Virginia, provides up-to-date information about immunizations, including reasons for being immunized, histories of specific immunizations, travel advisories, and news briefs.

Pan American Health Organization (PAHO)
<http://www.paho.org/>

PAHO is a part of the United Nations and is based in Washington, DC. The PAHO site includes current information, publications, and disease topics of interest to persons who travel overseas, especially to the Caribbean and South America.

☑ Vaccinations
<http://www.cdc.gov/travel/vaccinat.htm>

The U.S. Centers for Disease Control and Prevention (CDC) information about vaccinations includes travel vaccine recommendations for infants and children, vaccination requirements for yellow fever, information for immunocompromised travelers, and other material.

☑ Vaccine-Preventable Diseases
<http://www.who.int/ith/chapter06_01.html>

The World Health Organization (WHO) publishes *International Travel and Health*, which features a chapter on diseases that can be prevented by vaccines. The chapter covers vaccines for routine and selective use, mandatory vaccinations, special groups (children, frequent travelers, last-minute travelers, pregnant travelers), adverse reactions and contraindications, and documentation of vaccinations.

Vaccines in Pregnancy
<http://www.hon.ch/Dossier/MotherChild/preg_drugs/vaccines.html>

The Health on the Net (HON) Foundation's information about administration of live or inactive vaccines during pregnancy is derived from U.S. Centers for Disease Control and Prevention (CDC) information but is presented in an easily understood format.

☑ World Immunization Chart
<http://www.iamat.org/pdf/WorldImmunization.pdf>

Published by the International Association for Medical Assistance to Travellers (IAMAT) and frequently updated, this chart lists required and recommended immunizations for travel to specific countries; immunizations specific to travelers such as Muslim pilgrims and contract workers; and the geographic distribution of hepatitis B, Japanese encephalitis, rabies, plague, tick-borne encephalitis, and yellow fever (see Figure 3.2).

World Malaria Risk Chart
<http://www.iamat.org/pdf/WorldMalariaRisk.pdf>

Published by the International Association for Medical Assistance to Travellers (IAMAT) and frequently updated, this chart lists the relative risk of malaria in specific countries from

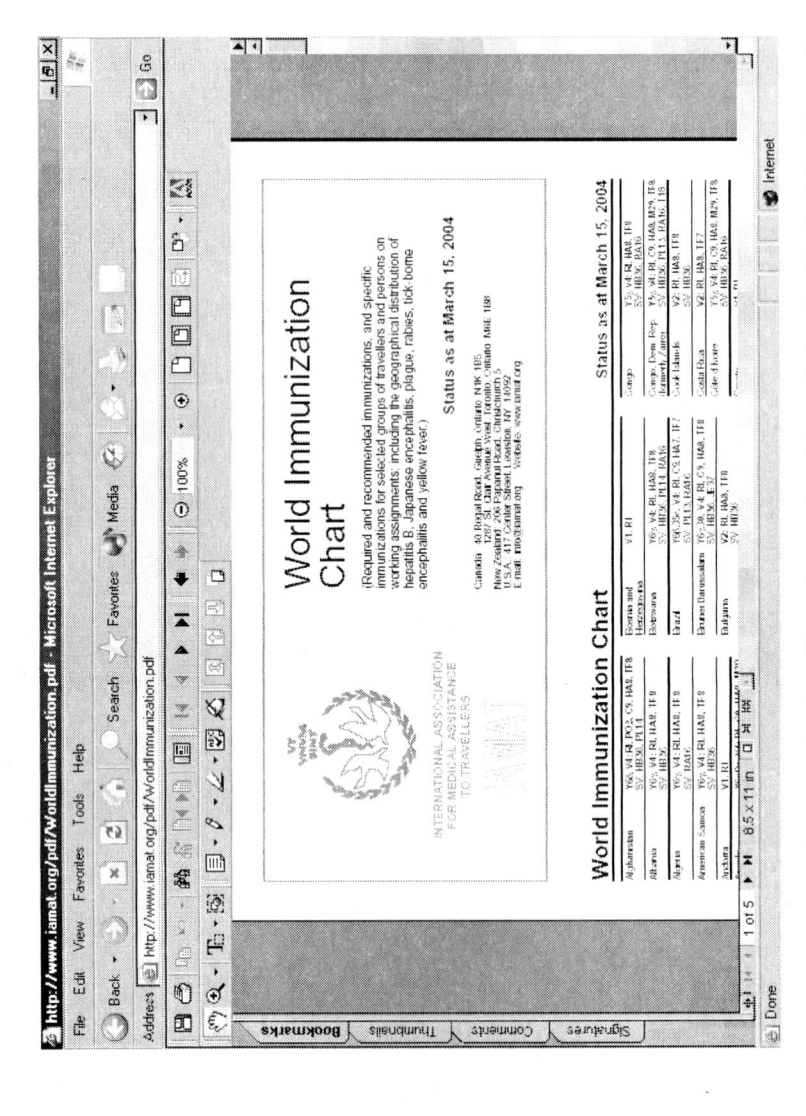

FIGURE 3.2. World Immunization Chart, International Association for Medical Assistance to Travellers (IAMAT) Web Site

Afghanistan to Zimbabwe and also includes a list of malaria-free countries.

MEDICATIONS, DEVICES, AND SUPPLIES

Checklist for Your Travel Medical Kit
<http://www.mydr.com.au/default.asp?article=2589>

MediMedia Australia publishes this site as well as drug reference texts and a journal, *Medical Observer*. The myDr.com.au site features a simple checklist for supplying a travel medical kit.

Flying with Diabetes
<http://www.childrenwithdiabetes.com/d_0j_211.htm>

Childrenwithdiabetes.com is an online community for children and families. The information about flying is based on advice from the Transportation Safety Administration (TSA) about carrying insulin, syringes, glucose meters, and other equipment through security checkpoints, with links to external sites related to carrying diabetes supplies while traveling.

Ostomy Supply Travel Certificate
<http://www.cmostomysupply.com/certificatetravel.htm>

The C&M Ostomy Supplies site features a form developed by the European Ostomy Association to assist persons with ostomies to travel with their ostomy supplies. The form explains the medical necessity of the supplies in a number of languages, including English, French, German, and Spanish.

Traveler's First Aid Kit
<http://www.mccg.org/adulthealth/travel/firstaid.asp>

The information on the Medical Center of Central Georgia (MCCG) site about supplying a travel first aid kit is based on recommendations made by the American College of Emergency Physicians (ACEP).

PREDEPARTURE HEALTH EXAMINATIONS

Pre-Travel Considerations
<http://www.hpechu.on.ca/Topics/PreTravel/preTravel Main.htm>

The Health Unit of Hastings and Prince Edward Counties in Ontario, Canada, has organized on its site information related to knowing and reducing travel risks, following a travel checklist, and obtaining pretravel immunizations.

Six to Eight Weeks Ahead
<http://www.healthatoz.com/healthatoz/Atoz/hl/sp/trvl/trasix.html>

HealthAtoZ.com developed this detailed advice for planning a healthy trip six to eight weeks before departure, including visiting a travel medicine clinic to receive the necessary immunizations, considering health insurance, and other information.

TRAVEL HEALTH INSURANCE

Global Travel Insurance
<http://www.globaltravelinsurance.com/>

Global Travel Insurance sells single and multiple trip travel medical insurance, covering "emergency evacuation, assistance, baggage, trip interruption coverage, optional hazardous sport coverage," and including a terrorism rider.

International Travel Insurance
<http://www.legendtravelers.com/>

Legend Travelers is a company that sells travel medical insurance for students, expatriate workers, and international citizens.

☑ Medical Information for Americans Traveling Abroad
<http://travel.state.gov/medical.html>

The U.S. State Department's travel site includes medical advice for Americans traveling or living abroad, including the high cost of medical evacuation, and the importance of carrying proof of insurance. The site also contains links to evacuation companies and travel insurance companies.

Medical Travel Insurance
<http://www.tripmedicalinsurance.com/>

Trip Medical Insurance.com sells short-term and long-term medical travel and trip cancellation insurance.

Travel Insurance and Assistance
<http://www.internationalsos.com/>

International SOS sells memberships providing emergency medical assistance and transportation for travelers.

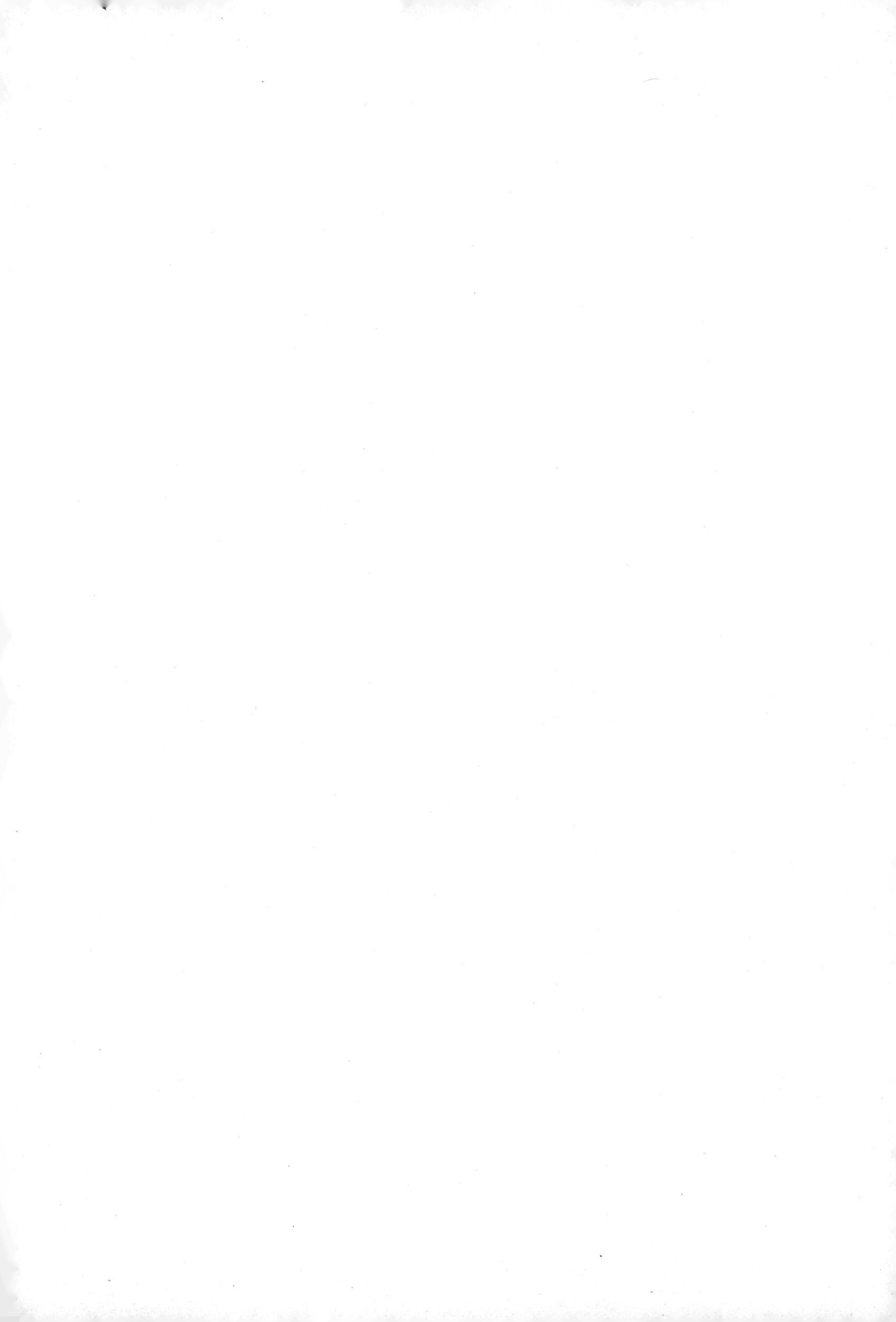

Chapter 4

Specific Issues and Concerns

This chapter covers specific issues and concerns of persons planning to travel, including traveling with children, seniors, and pets; traveling with disabilities; accident statistics; traveling by automobile, train, plane, bus, or ship; information about health tourism, which means traveling abroad for wellness, recuperation, or medical procedures such as cosmetic surgery; and researching weather forecasts prior to departure. The symbol ☑ is used to denote major resources that feature authoritative and original content.

ACCIDENTS

AAA Foundation for Traffic Safety
<http://www.aaafoundation.org/resources/>

The AAA Traffic Foundation for Traffic Safety works to prevent traffic accidents through educational outreach and research. The site includes online quizzes; educational materials about distracted driving, child safety seats, and drowsy driving; and other topics.

Major Airline Accidents by Country
<http://www.airsafe.com/events/regions/country.htm>

This commercial site provides information about air travel fatalities, including major airline accidents organized by country;

fear of flying; baggage limits; child safety; flight tracking; travel advisories; and other advice for passengers.

Road Safety Overseas
\<http://travel.state.gov/road_safety.html\>

The U.S. State Department provides up-to-date information about the relative risks of automobile travel in other countries, including road safety, road security, international driving permits, automobile insurance, as well as treaties on roads and transports. The site also contains links to reports on international road safety.

AUTOMOBILE TRAVEL

Driving Tips
\<http://www.aaroadwatch.ie/tips/\>

The Automobile Association of Ireland offers useful tips related to driving hazards in summer and winter, women driving alone, driving kits, route planning, and more.

FEMA Factsheet: Winter Driving Tips
\<http://www.fema.gov/hazards/winterstorms/winterf. shtm\>

The Federal Emergency Management Association (FEMA) is an independent agency of the U.S. government that focuses on disaster prevention, preparedness, and recovery. This fact sheet about winter driving provides useful information such as preparing a winter car kit and surviving a blizzard in a car.

Health and Travel Safety Tips
\<http://www.aaa-calif.com/travel/safety.asp\>

The Southern California chapter of the Automobile Club provides air and cruise travel tips and useful phone numbers.

Motor Vehicle Safety
<http://www.nlm.nih.gov/medlineplus/motorvehiclesafety.html>

MedlinePlus organizes content and links about motor vehicle safety, including the latest news, general overviews, prevention and screening, research, specific conditions and aspects, directories, law and policy, organizations, statistics, and more.

National Scenic Byways
<http://www.byways.org/>

This site is maintained by the Federal Highway Administration of the U.S. Department of Transportation (DOT). Features include maps, weather information, and pictures of value to travelers in the United States.

☑ *Physician's Guide to Assessing and Counseling Older Drivers*
<http://www.ama-assn.org/ama/pub/category/10791.html/>

The American Medical Association (AMA) issued this guide for physicians to assess an individual's medical fitness to drive, including possible conditions and medications that can affect driving ability and strategies to counsel patients suspected of being unsafe drivers (see Figure 4.1).

☑ Road Safety Overseas
<http://travel.state.gov/road_safety.html>

American Citizen Services of the Bureau of Consular Affairs of the U.S. Department of State provides information about road safety, road security, international driving permits, automobile insurance, driving in other countries, as well as treaties on roads and transport. The site also contains links to other sites.

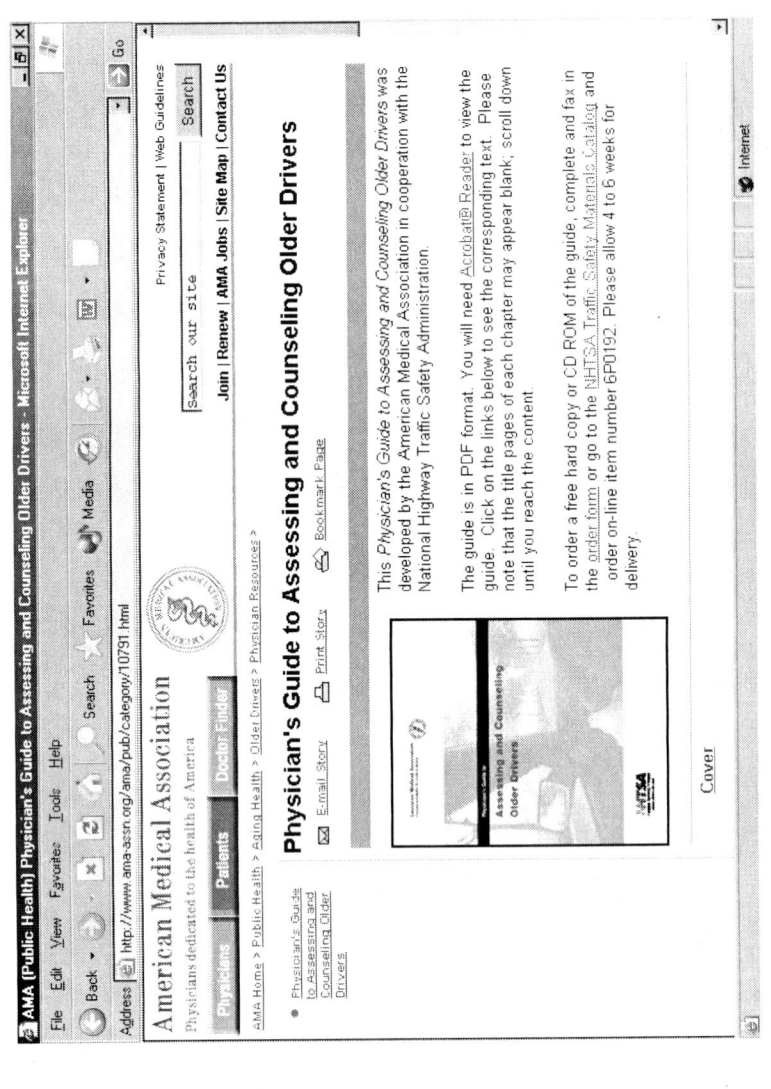

FIGURE 4.1. *Physician's Guide to Assessing and Counseling Older Drivers*, American Medical Association (AMA) Web Site

BUS OR TRAIN TRAVEL

How Safe Are the Railways?
<http://www.hse.gov.uk/railways/howsafe.htm>

The Health Safety Commission (HSC) and Health Safety Executive (HSE) regulate work health and safety in the United Kingdom. The HSE site includes information about railroad safety, rail passenger fatalities from 1975 to 2002, and rail accident reports.

Operation Lifesaver
<http://www.oli.org/>

Operation Lifesaver is a nonprofit organization devoted to reducing train collisions and improving public awareness of safety issues near railroad crossings. The site features information for teachers, students, law enforcement, and the media. Although primarily related to railroad crossing, persons who travel by train may be interested in the railroad crossing injury statistics and other information.

Rail Transportation Abroad
<http://travel.state.gov/rail_transport.html>

The U.S. State Department's site organizes links useful to persons planning to travel by rail in the United States, Canada, or the United Kingdom.

Traveling by Train or Bus
<http://www.pueblo.gsa.gov/links/th5links.htm>

The Federal Citizen Information Center in Pueblo, Colorado, provides free, practical consumer information through this site and its catalog of publications. The information specific to traveling by train or bus includes annotated links to government transit and transportation organizations, and private sector bus and train companies such as Amtrak, Britrail, Eurostar, Greyhound, etc.

CHILDREN TRAVELING ALONE AND TRAVELING WITH CHILDREN

Children Traveling Alone
<http://www.airgorilla.com/help/childalone.html>

AirGorilla, a site that focuses on discount fares and travel reservations, also aggregates links to policies related to children traveling alone on the major airlines.

Health on the Road
<http://www.familytravelguides.com/articles/health/index.html>

Organized into four parts, this information is derived from *Lonely Planet Travel with Children,* Fourth Edition (Lonely Planet Publications, 2002), written by Cathy Lanigan and Maureen Wheeler. Although the content focuses on children, other useful information includes medical kits, medical treatment, avoiding jet lag, various infectious diseases, insect-borne diseases, and more.

Kids Traveling Tips
<http://www.freetraveltips.com/Kids/Kids07.htm>

Although the Free Travel Tips site primarily offers online booking of airline and hotel reservations, the site also includes helpful tips for parents of children traveling alone on airplanes.

Plan Your Child's Solo Journey by Bus
<http://familyfun.go.com/travel/places/feature/dony37solobus/dony37solobus.html>

This information is part of DisneyOnline's FamilyFun site. The section about children traveling alone by bus includes common bus procedures.

Specific Issues and Concerns 41

Plan Your Child's Solo Journey by Plane
<http://familyfun.go.com/travel/places/feature/dony37solo plane/dony37soloplane.html>

Also included on DisneyOnline's FamilyFun site, this section about children traveling alone by plane includes common airline procedures.

Plan Your Child's Solo Train Trip
<http://familyfun.go.com/travel/places/feature/dony37solo train/dony37solotrain.html>

Another part of DisneyOnline's FamilyFun site, this section about children traveling alone by train includes common train procedures.

Top Ten Safety Tips for Children Traveling Alone
<http://www.airsafe.com/kidsafe/kidsolo.htm>

This commercial site offers practical advice for children traveling alone, including reviewing airline policies, explaining the journey to the child, and spending extra time at the airport.

Travelling with Children
<http://www.travellingwithchildren.co.uk>

Travellingwithchildren.co.uk is a British-based site that focuses on general information for traveling with children by foot, train, ship, and plane.

VIA Rail Canada/Children Travelling Alone
<http://www.viarail.ca/families/en_fami_enfa_noac.html>

VIA Rail Canada is an independent crown corporation, meaning a corporation established by the Canadian government. The site features information of interest to families traveling by train and to children traveling alone by train.

CONTRAINDICATIONS TO TRAVEL

☑ Medical Contraindications for Air Travel
<http://www.aviation-health.org/guidelines_for_gps.html>

The Aviation Health Institute is a charity organization based in the United Kingdom (see Figure 4.2). Areas of interest include preventing a variety of aviation-related conditions, including deep vein thrombosis and radiation. Contraindications to air travel include specific conditions and surgical procedures.

Medical Contraindications to Air Travel
<http://www.listermedicalcentre.com/travel_advice.htm#ci>

The Lister Medical Centre in Essex, England, lists a number of medical conditions that can be affected adversely by airplane travel.

Travel and Avoiding Dizziness
<http://www.dizziness-and-balance.com/treatment/flying.html>

Dr. Timothy C. Hain, an otolaryngologist (ear, nose, and throat specialist) associated with Northwestern University Medical School in Chicago, Illinois, discusses specific conditions that cause dizziness and may be worsened by airplane travel.

Traveling When Sick
<http://www.skylarkmedicalclinic.com/sick.html>

Skylark Medical Clinic, located in Winnipeg, Manitoba, Canada, covers a number of health conditions that contraindicate travel.

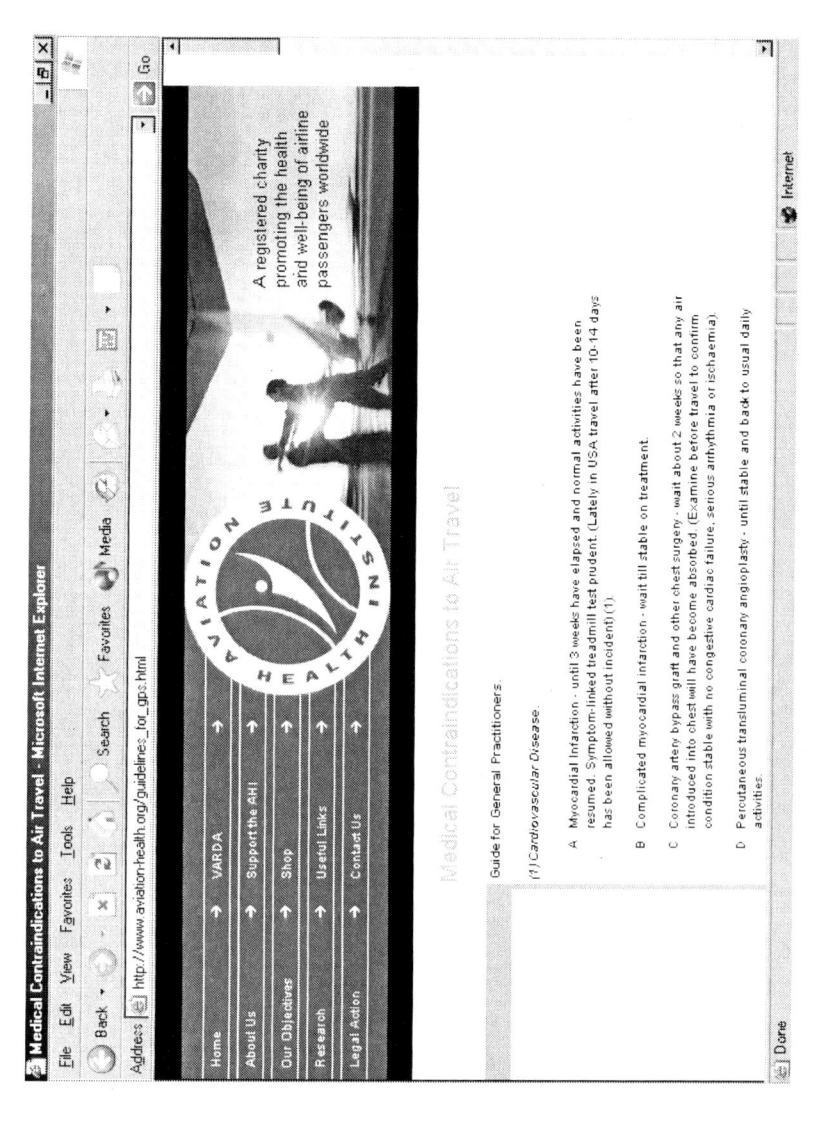

FIGURE 4.2. Medical Contraindications to Air Travel, Aviation Health Institute Web Site

CRUISE SHIP TRAVEL

Cruise Lines and Ship Accessibility
<http://www.access-able.com/dbase/cruise.cfm>

Access-Able Travel Source lists contact information by cruise ship line.

☑ Cruise Ship Travel
<http://www.cdc.gov/travel/cruise.htm> and
<http://www.cdc.gov/travel/cruiships.htm>

The U.S. Centers for Disease Control and Prevention (CDC) site includes two sections about the risks of cruise travel. Precautions and preventive measures depend on the destinations visited, but the site also covers basic sanitation measures, health recommendations, and information about vessel sanitation and inspections.

Cruising with Confidence
<http://www.fda.gov/fdac/features/2003/303_virus.html>

The U.S. Food and Drug Administration (FDA) provides information about preventing gastroenteritis (stomach or intestinal upset) while taking a cruise.

Sanitation Inspections of International Cruise Ships
<http://www2.cdc.gov/nceh/vsp/vspmain.asp>

The U.S. Centers for Disease Control and Prevention (CDC) publishes *Summary of Sanitation Inspections of International Cruise Ships,* also known as the "Green Sheet." This publication lists ships by name, inspection date, and score. Sanitation standards cover water; food preparation and holding; potential contamination of food; and general cleanliness, storage, and repair.

DEATH

Consular Report of Death of a U.S. Citizen Abroad
<http://travel.state.gov/deathrep.html>

This page describes the procedures to follow to get a valid death certificate if an American dies outside of the United States.

Fatality Facts
<http://www.hwysafety.org/safety_facts/safety.htm>

The Insurance Institute for Highway Safety has conducted research since 1969 on the human, vehicular, and environmental factors that cause motor vehicle crashes. This site features information about vehicle ratings; injury, collision, and theft losses by vehicle make and model; state law facts; and recent fatality statistics according to involvement with pedestrians, bicycles, large trucks, motorcycles, alcohol, roadside hazards, etc.

DISABILITIES

Access-Able Travel Source
<http://www.access-able.com/>

Access-Able Travel Source has offered useful information for older and/or disabled travelers since 1995. Useful features include detailed information (accommodations, equipment rental, transportation, attractions, adventures, access guides, etc.) for accessible world destinations for travelers and travel agents, cruise ship accessibility information, and more.

Disability Link Barn
<http://www.accessunlimited.com/links.html>

Access Unlimited, based in Binghamton, New York, manufactures and distributes mobility equipment, including lift seats, clutch systems, and control systems to help the disabled drive automobiles. The site's Disability Link Barn includes useful travel links related to airlines, accessible accommodations and destinations, and more.

Fodor's—Disabilities and Accessibility
<http://www.fodors.com/traveltips/disabilities/>

Fodor's publishes the well-known travel guide series. This site features information of interest to travelers with disabilities, including general information about the Americans with Disabilities Act (ADA); insurance, lodging, and transportation (airplane, bus, automobile, train); travel agencies that cater to the disabled; as well as links to similar sites.

Gimp on the Go
<http://gimponthego.com/>

Despite the insensitive name, this site is maintained by a disabled individual who explains that the term *gimp* is used to "establish a candid atmosphere." The site includes travel reviews, bulletin boards, surveys, a searchable database of accessible destinations, and more.

Handicapped Travel Club
<http://www.handicappedtravelclub.com/>

The Handicapped Travel Club (HTC) focuses on making travel by recreational vehicle (RV) more accessible to persons with disabilities. The HTC site includes annotated links, campground information, a campground criteria checklist, and more.

Minnesota Travel Guide for Persons with Disabilities
<http://www.accessminnesota.org/>

Access for All developed this travel guide that covers Minnesota lodging, restaurants, amusement parks, resorts, nightclubs, historic sites, convention centers, transportation, campgrounds, etc., equipped for persons with disabilities.

New Horizons: Information for the Air Traveler with a Disability
<http://www.faa.gov/acr/dat.htm> and <http://airconsumer.ost.dot.gov/publications/horizons.htm>

The U.S. Federal Aviation Administration's Office of Civil Rights provides advice and tips for disabled air travelers, including trip planning, getting on and off the plane, service animals, in-cabin service, and other information.

Passengers with Disabilities
<http://airconsumer.ost.dot.gov/publications/disabled.htm>

The Aviation Consumer Protection Division of the U.S. Department of Transportation (DOT) site excerpts pertinent sections of the Air Carrier Access Act (Title 14, *Code of Federal Regulations*, Part 382), which refers to U.S. airlines accommodating passengers with disabilities.

Project ACTION Accessible Traveler's Database
<http://www.projectaction.easterseals.com/cgi=bin/traveler_search.cgi>

The Project ACTION Accessible Traveler's Database provides information about public transit operators, accessible van rental companies, private bus/tour companies with accessible vehicles, accessible taxicabs, accessible airport transportation at selected airports, and more. The database is searchable by state and city.

The Savvy Traveler—Disability Resources
<http://savvy.mpr.org/before/disability-resource.shtml>

The Savvy Traveler is a public radio travel program and Web site hosted by athlete and journalist Diana Nyad. The site provides information for disabled travelers, including contact information (address, phone number) for relevant organizations, helpful tips, suggested reading, and more.

EVACUATION SERVICES

Evacuation II—Safety Tips for Emergency Travel
<http://disaster.ifas.ufl.edu/PDFS/CHAP03/D03-04.PDF>

The Cooperative Extension Service of the University of Florida prepared this evacuation safety sheet, including tips for evacuating an area by automobile.

International SOS
<http://www.intsos.com/>

International SOS is a company that sells short-term and long-term evacuation coverage and travel insurance.

Medical Evacuation
<http://www.travdoc.com/articles/art14.html>

TravDoc is a travel clinic located in Michigan. One of the site's articles discusses aspects of being evacuated for medical reasons.

☑ Medical Information for Americans Traveling Abroad
<http://travel.state.gov/medical.html>

The U.S. Department of State recommends that American citizens take their insurance cards and claim forms with them when traveling to other countries and warns that medical evacuation can be costly. This page lists a number of U.S.- and foreign-based air ambulance and medical evacuation companies.

MEDJET Assistance
<http://www.medjetassistance.com/>

MEDJET Assistance sells individual and family memberships for emergency evacuation services.

HEALTH TOURISM

Cosmetic Surgery Vacations
<http://lorrypatton.com/travel/gtips/2882.html>

Travel Tips 'n' Tales is an online travel magazine published by travel writer Lorry Patton. The information on cosmetic surgery vacations is practical and thought-provoking.

European Healthnet: Surgery Abroad
<http://www.surgeryabroad.net/faq.htm>

European Healthnet serves as a clearinghouse of information for persons seeking surgery abroad. The site sells a brochure that describes orthopaedic, eye, cosmetic, and other surgeries available in various European countries (France, Belgium, Germany, Ireland, Switzerland, and Spain) as well as in India, Russia, Poland, Costa Rica, and Cuba. The site also includes useful information about typical prices for such procedures as knee replacement, breast enlargement, cataract surgery, etc., and frequently asked questions about seeking treatments abroad.

International Medical Services
<http://www.medicaltrips.com/terms.htm>

International Medical Services (IMS) is a company that arranges surgery and medical procedures to be performed in Kaunas, Lithuania.

Surgeon and Safari
<http://www.surgeon-and-safari.co.za/>

Surgeon and Safari is a South African organization that arranges and offers surgical procedures, recuperation, spa treatments, and safari tours.

Surgitours
<http://www.surgitours.co.za/>

Surgitours is a South African-based company that arranges and offers surgical procedures, recuperation, and travel tours.

MEDICAL CARE WHILE TRAVELING

Health and Illness Overseas
<http://www.familytravelguides.com/articles/health/illabrod.html>

FamilyTravelGuides is a site that offers tips for preventing and treating illnesses while traveling overseas, including overcoming jet lag, traveling with children, and preventing specific travel-related conditions.

☑ Illness Abroad
<http://www.cdc.gov/travel/other/illness-abroad.htm>

The National Center for Infectious Diseases maintains travel health content on the U.S. Centers for Disease Control and Prevention (CDC) site. The information about preparing for medical emergencies while traveling includes seeking medical care while abroad, contacting a consular officer, understanding World Health Organization (WHO) blood transfusion guidelines, procedures for reporting a death overseas, and diseases that may manifest themselves long after the international trip.

In-Flight Medicine: Handling Illness at 30,000 Feet
<http://www.mayoclinic.com/invoke.cfm?id=WL00027>

The Mayo Clinic offers advice for handling medical emergencies that present themselves during airplane flight and discusses some conditions that may cause discomfort or problems during flight.

☑ Medical Information for Americans Traveling Abroad
<http://travel.state.gov/medical.html>

The U.S. Department of State recommends that American citizens take their insurance cards and claim forms with them when traveling to other countries and warns that medical evacuation can be costly. This page lists a number of U.S.- and foreign-based air ambulance and medical evacuation companies.

MEDICATIONS

☑ Customs and Border Protection—Medication/Drugs
<http://www.customs.gov/xp/cgov/travel/alerts/medication_drugs.xml>

The U.S. Department of Homeland Security details the regulations related to carrying medications in and out of the United States.

Drugs and Travel
<http://www.voyage.gc.ca/main/drugs_menu-en.asp>

Canada's Department of Foreign Affairs and International Trade offers advice about carrying medical supplies while traveling, relates stories of Canadians imprisoned for smuggling illegal drugs, and explains judicial systems outside of Canada.

Purchasing Medications Outside the United States
<http://www.fda.gov/ora/import/purchasing_medications.htm>

The U.S. Food and Drug Administration (FDA) warns that some medications purchased abroad can have significant health risks.

Safe Traveling Tips
<http://www.travelsense.org/tips/healthsafety.sp>

The American Society of Travel Agents (ASTA) offers travel tips, including the dangers of carrying illegal drugs while traveling.

Travel Smart with Medications
<http://www.roadandtravel.com/health/travelmedications.htm>

The American Woman Road & Travel site features information about traveling with medications. This resource is a companion site to *American Woman Road & Travel* magazine.

NATURAL DISASTERS

☑ Crisis Awareness and Preparedness
<http://travel.state.gov/crisismg.html>

The U.S. Department of State's Bureau of Consular Affairs has organized a list of links useful to persons interested in monitoring crisis situations and disasters overseas, including earthquakes, fires, floods, hurricanes, typhoons, tsunamis, thunderstorms, heat waves, winter storms, evacuations, terrorism, and other concerns.

Travel Intelligence—Disaster Travel
<http://www.travelintelligence.net/wsd/category/cat_44.html>

Travel Intelligence features the work of more than seventy travel writers. Essays include traveling to disaster areas and disastrous experiences during trips.

PETS TRAVELING ALONE AND TRAVELING WITH PETS

Advance Planning Eases Travel with Pets
<http://www.seniorsgotravel.com/general/safePets.html>

The Seniors Go Travel.com site features information about traveling with pets that emphasizes advance planning when traveling by automobile or airplane.

Air Travel Tips—ASPCA
<http://www.aspca.org/site/PageServer?pagename=travel tips>

The American Society for the Prevention of Cruelty to Animals (ASPCA) site includes tips for preparing pets for travel (checkup, health certificate, shipping crate, etc.).

Dogs in the Family: Travel Tips
<http://www.akc.org/life/family/vac_hols/travel_tips.cfm>

The American Kennel Club (AKC) gives useful information about traveling with dogs by automobile, plane, train, boat, or bus; suggested publications; and other information.

The Flying Dog
<http://www.bellaonline.com/articles/art3785.asp>

BellaOnline is a site that focuses on women, including information channels about education, careers, beauty, hobbies, travel, and more. The site's travel channel discusses flying with dogs. Annotated links to other sites include consolidated information about airline pet travel policies.

Fodor's: Pets and Travel
<http://www.fodors.com/traveltips/pets/>

Fodor's publishes the well-known travel guide series. This site features information of interest to persons traveling with pets, including making sure the pet is travel-ready, preparing or training pets to travel, and finding pet-friendly accommodations. The site also provides annotated links to other resources.

Independent Pet and Animal Transportation Association (IPATA) International
<http://www.ipata.com>

Members of this organization include animal handlers, pet moving providers, kennel operators, veterinarians, and others. The site features answers to frequently asked questions (FAQs). The list of pet shippers is organized by company name or location.

International Travel with Your Dog
<http://petplace.netscape.com/articles/artShow.asp?artID=2621>

PetPlace.com features expert information from veterinarians about pet health. The section about traveling to international destinations with a dog covers health certificate and quarantine requirements for ten specific countries.

InterPet Explorer
<http://www.interpetexplorer.com/>

InterPet Explorer is a commercial site focusing on pet-friendly hotels, pet sitters, and traveling with pets. The searchable interface and clickable map yield state-specific pet sitters and pet-friendly accommodations. Travel topics include avoiding travel sickness, guidelines for driving with dogs, and air travel with dogs.

Pet Air Travel
<http://www.aimrelocation.com/pettravel/air.html>

AIM Relocation is a site devoted to national and international relocations with details about shipping pets to domestic and foreign locations. Useful features include a traveling pet checklist, airline requirements, import guidelines, and other information.

Pet Chauffeur
<http://www.petride.com/>

This commercial pet transportation company sells food, accessories, supplies, and transportation services for a full range of pets, including dogs, cats, birds, fish, hamsters, ferrets, reptiles, etc.

Pet Travel
<http://www.aimrelocation.com/pettravel/>

This pet travel information is provided by AIM Relocation, a relocation firm. Information includes a pet travel checklist, automobile travel, air travel, pet-friendly hotels, and relocating to international destinations with pets. Some information is specific to the type of pet, such as dog, cat, bird or other caged pet, tropical fish, and horses.

Pets on the Go
<http://www.petsonthego.com/>

Dawbert Press, Inc., maintains this site that focuses on pet travel, including pet-friendly accommodations, pet emergencies, determining if a specific pet is suitable for travel, entry requirements for specific countries, expert pet travel advice, a members-only discussion forum, and other information.

Preparation for a Road Trip
<http://www.dogfriendly.com/server/travel/info/tips/plan.shtml>

DogFriendly.com publishes "nationwide city guides and travel guides for dog owners." The site features dog-friendly lodging, attractions, and preparation tips for road trips.

Takeyourpet.com
<http://www.takeyourpet.com/>

Although this site is restricted to subscribers only, the membership fee is minimal. Members are entitled to discounts on pet-friendly accommodations; information about pet-sitting services, pet food, and veterinarians in specific cities; and a members-only discussion board.

Transporting Live Animals
<http://airconsumer.ost.dot.gov/publications/animals.htm>

The U.S. Department of Transportation's Aviation Consumer Protection Division details aspects of the Federal Animal Welfare Act as applied to transporting live animals.

Traveling by Car with Your Pet
<http://www.healthypet.com/Library/petcare-30.html>

The American Animal Hospital Association (AAHA) maintains the HealthyPet.com site, which features car travel tips in its pet care library.

The Traveling Dog
<http://www.bellaonline.com/subjects/567.asp>

BellaOnline is a site dedicated to collecting and organizing content of interest and value to women. The site's seventeen channels include beauty and self, entertainment, news and politics, travel and leisure, and more. The travel and leisure channel includes annotated links about vacation pet care, camping with dogs, dog-friendly accommodations, and pet safety.

Traveling with Pets
<http://www.state.gov/m/fsi/tc/1870.htm>

The U.S. State Department explains the procedures for entering the United States with pets, including confirming entry requirements and obtaining U.S. Department of Agriculture (USDA) certificates. The site also provides a checklist for shipping pets.

Traveling with Pets
<http://www.travelsense.org/tips/pets.asp>

The American Society of Travel Agents (ASTA) offers tips for traveling with pets, including pretravel checkups, airline limitations, travel kennels, and links to some external sites.

Traveling with Your Cat or Kitten
<http://www.cat-on-board.com/>

The Cat-on-Board.com site focuses on three areas of concern for persons planning to travel with felines: getting ready, cat carriers, and travel litter box supplies.

Traveling with Your Pet
<http://www.aphis.usda.gov/oa/pubs/petravel.html>

The Animal and Plant Health Inspection Service (APHIS) of the U.S. Department of Agriculture (USDA) provides advice about planning trips with animals, including the minimum age for cats and dogs (eight weeks and weaned), kennels, feeding and watering during transit, traveling with birds, and other hints (see Figure 4.3).

Traveling with Your Pet
<http://www.avma.org/careforanimals/animatedjourneys/livingwithpets/traveling.asp>

The American Veterinary Medical Association (AVMA) accredits veterinary medical schools in the United States and Canada. AVMA's site includes useful information for traveling with pets, including trip planning; camping; and travel by automobile, bus, train, or airplane.

United States Department of Agriculture
Animal and Plant Health Inspection Service

Traveling With Your Pet

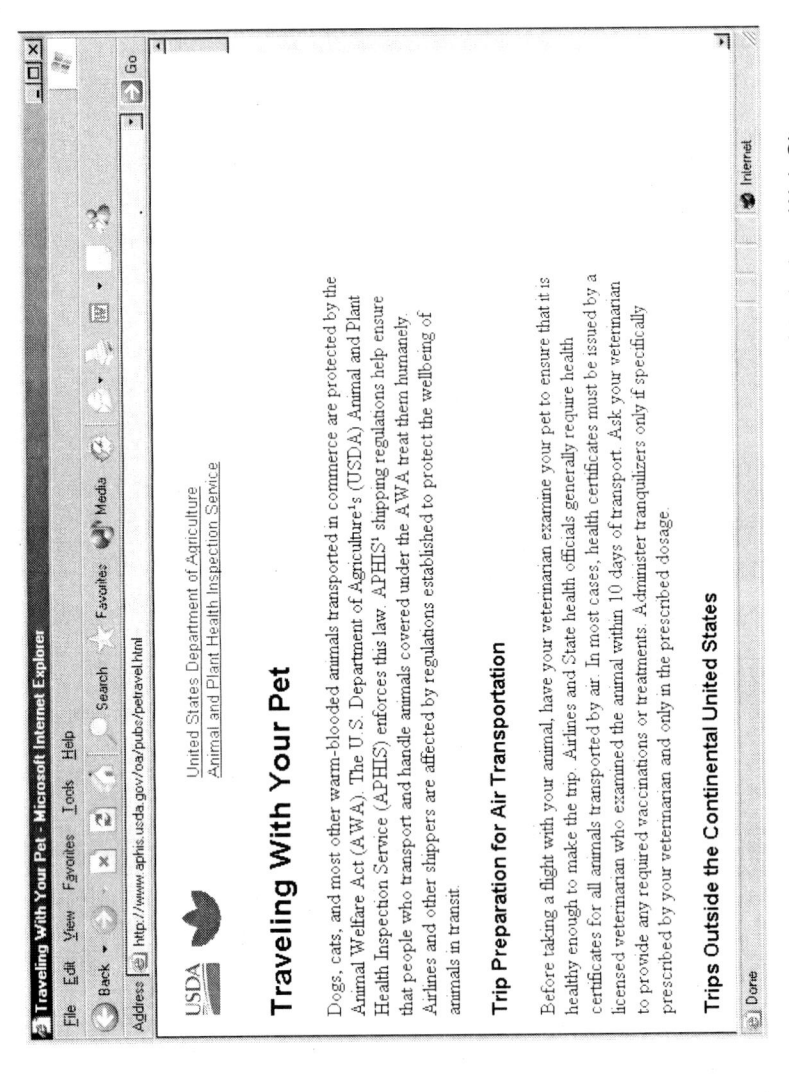

Dogs, cats, and most other warm-blooded animals transported in commerce are protected by the Animal Welfare Act (AWA). The U.S. Department of Agriculture's (USDA) Animal and Plant Health Inspection Service (APHIS) enforces this law. APHIS' shipping regulations help ensure that people who transport and handle animals covered under the AWA treat them humanely. Airlines and other shippers are affected by regulations established to protect the wellbeing of animals in transit.

Trip Preparation for Air Transportation

Before taking a flight with your animal, have your veterinarian examine your pet to ensure that it is healthy enough to make the trip. Airlines and State health officials generally require health certificates for all animals transported by air. In most cases, health certificates must be issued by a licensed veterinarian who examined the animal within 10 days of transport. Ask your veterinarian to provide any required vaccinations or treatments. Administer tranquilizers only if specifically prescribed by your veterinarian and only in the prescribed dosage.

Trips Outside the Continental United States

FIGURE 4.3. Traveling with Your Pet, U.S. Department of Agriculture Web Site

Specific Issues and Concerns 59

QUARANTINE

Australian Quarantine and Inspection Services (AQIS)
<http://www.affa.gov.au/>

AQIS inspects passengers, animals, plants, and cargo that enter Australia. This site includes news headlines, hot topics, and advice about importing flora and fauna.

☑ Bringing Pets to Britain
<http://www.defra.gov.uk/animalh/quarantine/index.htm>

The United Kingdom's Department for Environment, Food and Rural Affairs (DEFRA) administers rabies import controls. Britain's Pet Travel Scheme (PETS) covers cats and dogs entering the United Kingdom by air, sea, and train. As long as specific rules are met, cats and dogs from certain countries can enter the United Kingdom without quarantine.

Dogs, Cats, Pets, People, Property
<http://www.familysafety.com/travel/international/interna.shtml>

Family Safety Solutions, LLC, sells a pet ID tag and maintains a commercial site called Family Safety. The information about traveling with or without pets includes quarantine, pet-friendly lodging, automobile travel, pets as air cargo or in the cabin, preparing pets for moving, and other topics.

Human Quarantine
<http://www.health.gov.au/pubhlth/strateg/quaranti/>

The Australian Department of Health and Ageing site features useful information about quarantine arrangements, vaccination requirements, travel health advice, and travel health risks within Australia.

Overseas Pet Quarantine Regulations
  <http://www.sniksnak.com/quarantine.html>

Although this pet quarantine information for specific destinations (Bahrain, Guam, Hawaii, Italy, Japan, etc.) is intended for U.S. Navy personnel, others may find the information useful.

Pet Import for Animals Travelling to the UK
  <http://www.airpets.com/arrivals_home.html>

AirPets Oceanic is a pet boarding company located near Heathrow Airport. The AirPets site includes information about entering the United Kingdom with pets, boarding animals at the AirPets kennels, travel containers, and other information.

SENIORS TRAVELING ALONE AND TRAVELING WITH SENIORS

Elderly Travellers
  <http://www.fitfortravel.scot.nhs.uk/General/Elderly.html>

Developed by the Travel Medicine Division at the Scottish Centre for Infection and Environmental Health (SCIEH), the Fitfortravel site includes concise, practical information for older travelers, including pretravel medical assessment, travel insurance, skin and foot care, vaccinations, and malaria prevention.

☑ **FirstGov for Seniors—Travel and Leisure**
  <http://www.firstgov.gov/Topics/Seniors.shtml>

FirstGov for Seniors, a site maintained by the U.S. Social Security Administration, provides an aggregated portal to all U.S. government sites of potential interest to senior citizens (see Figure 4.4). The information about travel features links to government sites about disease prevention, customs, currency exchange rates, U.S. State Department travel advisories, weather, and more.

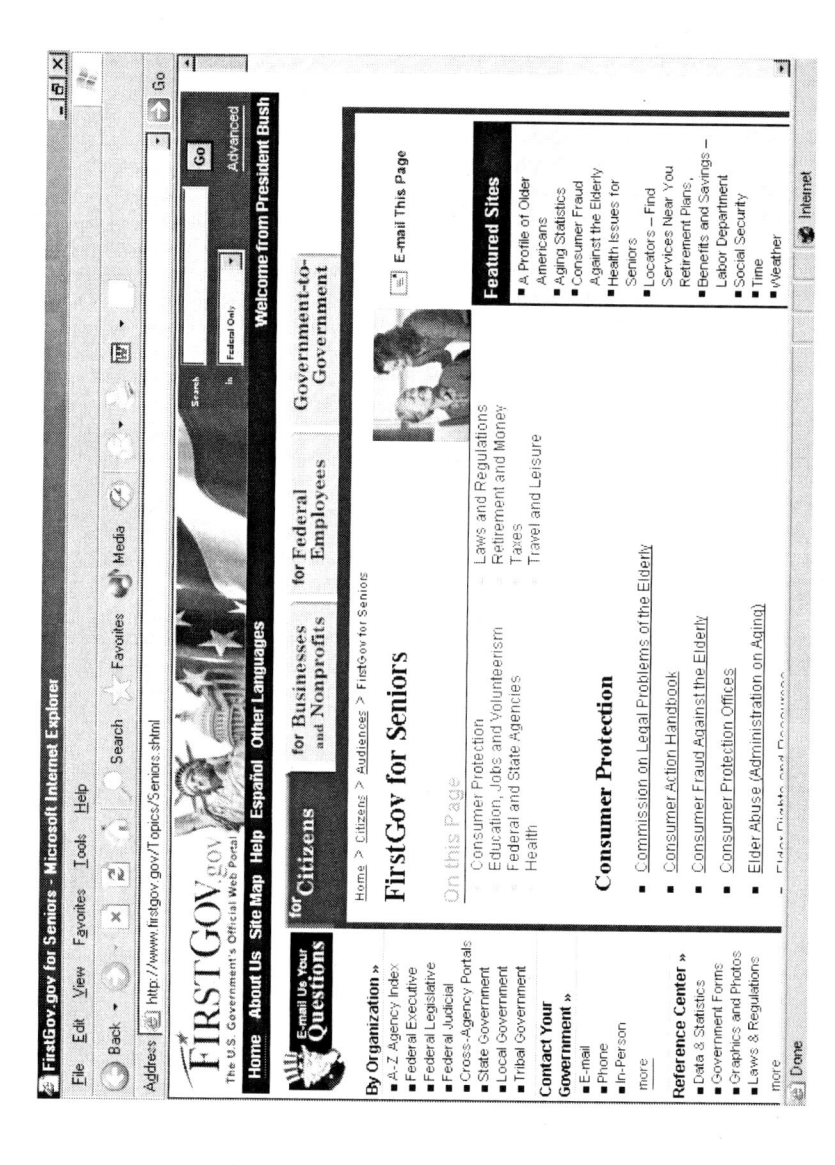

FIGURE 4.4. Travel and Leisure, FirstGov for Seniors Web Site

61

Seniors and Traveling
<http://www.ahealthyme.com/topic/srtravel>

HealthyMe is a site maintained by BlueCross BlueShield of Massachusetts. The information about senior travelers covers staying in hostels; taking day trips; traveling alone; and taking bus, ship, walking, or bicycle tours.

WEATHER

Weather Forecasts by City and State
<http://www.wrh.noaa.gov/wrhq/nwspage.html>

The National Weather Service site of the U.S. National Oceanic and Atmospheric Administration (NOAA) site includes city-specific forecasts and past weather information.

Weather Warnings/Advisories
<http://weather.gov/>

The National Weather Service of the U.S. National Oceanic and Atmospheric Administration (NOAA) provides weather warning and advisory information of interest to persons planning to travel by air, boat, or motor vehicle.

Yahoo! Weather
<http://weather.yahoo.com/>

Yahoo! provides a weather interface, searchable by city or zip code, or browsable by broad geographic area, such as Asia, Central America, Pacific Rim, etc. Typical city-specific information includes current temperature, daily high and low temperatures, five-day forecasts, humidity, visibility, wind speed and direction, dew point, time of sunrise, time of sunset, and more.

WOMEN TRAVELING ALONE

Female Travellers
<http://www.travelhealth.co.uk/advice/female.htm>

The TravelHealth.co.uk site provides advice to women traveling alone, including safety, security, and personal health issues.

Tips for Women Traveling Alone
<http://travel.state.gov/tips_women.html>

The U.S. State Department site includes useful tips for women traveling alone, including trip preparation (passports, visas, health coverage, clothing), and links to external sites.

Chapter 5

Diseases, Conditions, and Ailments

This chapter includes links of interest to persons diagnosed with specific diseases, conditions, and ailments as well as information about preventing other conditions that may be encountered while traveling. The symbol ☑ is used to denote major resources with authoritative and original content.

AIR RAGE AND ROAD RAGE

Accident Reconstruction Research: Avoiding Road Rage
  <http://www.accidentreconstruction.com/research/road rage/index.asp>

The accident reconstruction network site (arcNetwork) features information about recognizing, avoiding, and reducing the risks of road rage, as well as annotated links to external sites dealing with the subject.

Air Rage Information Sources
  <http://www.airsafe.com/issues/rage.htm>

This commercial site features links to organizations devoted to the subject of air rage, media coverage of air rage incidents, suggested books on the subject, air rage statistics from 1995 onward, and filing complaints.

65

Air Rage Prevention
<http://www.drdriving.org/rages/>

Drs. Leon James and Diane Nahl are the experts who provide content for the drdriving.org site. Featured information covers a variety of rages, including air, road, sky, surf, shopping, and parking; surveys and tests; and anecdotes.

Avoiding Road Rage on the Highways
<http://www.homeandawaymagazine.com/1824.cfm>

Michael D. Lee, an instructor with the National Safety Council and author of a book about road rage, offers information about recognizing aggressive driving behaviors and eight tips for avoiding road rage.

The Skyrage Foundation
<http://www.skyrage.org/ragepage2.html>

The Skyrage Foundation is based in Summerville, South Carolina. The site includes editorials, headlines, and research related to this topic.

ALLERGIES AND ASTHMA

Anaphylaxis Campaign
<http://www.anaphylaxis.org.uk/air.html>

The United Kingdom's Anaphylaxis Campaign provides up-to-date information for persons with life-threatening allergies, including food alerts and airlines that have agreed to remove peanut products from their meals.

Anaphylaxis Canada: Safe Travel
<http://www.anaphylaxis.org/content/programs/programs_advocacy_travel.asp>

Anaphylaxis Canada is an organization dedicated to providing authoritative information about severe allergic reactions. Air travel safety tips include preventing in-flight reactions.

Flying with a Peanut Allergy
<http://www.foodallergy.org/topics_archive/flying.html>

This information, developed by the Food Allergy and Anaphylaxis Network (FAAN), will be helpful for persons sensitive to peanuts and peanut-based foods.

Food Allergies and Travel
<http://edition.cnn.com/HEALTH/library/HQ/00709.html>

This information, updated in 2002, is hosted on the CNN.com site but was developed by MayoClinic.com. Tips include symptoms of allergic reactions, allergy tests, the dangers of air travel for persons with peanut allergies, and packing for emergencies.

Travel and Asthma
<http://www.asthma.co.za/articles/ref04.htm>

South Africa's National Asthma Education Programme site includes information about travel and asthma written by a physician.

Travel for Kids: Allergies Abroad
<http://www.travelforkids.com/Travelessentials/allergies.htm>

Travel for Kids is a commercial site that relies on first-person accounts of the joys and challenges of traveling with children. The information about traveling with allergies covers the most common allergies (dairy, eggs, nuts, peanuts, shellfish, soybeans, and wheat), symptoms, and preparation.

Traveling with Allergies and Asthma
<http://www.aaaai.org/patients/publicedmat/tips/travelingwithallergies.stm>

The American Academy of Allergy, Asthma, and Immunology (AAAAI) provides authoritative allergy information for persons planning to travel by automobile, bus, train, plane, or ship.

ALTITUDE SICKNESS

CIWEC Clinic Travel Medicine Center—Altitude Illness
<http://www.ciwec-clinic.com/altitude/>

The CIWEC Clinical Travel Medicine Center is located in Kathmandu, Nepal. This site includes information about the symptoms, prevention, and treatment of altitude sickness.

High Altitude Medicine Guide
<http://www.high-altitude-medicine.com/>

This guide was developed by Thomas E. Dietz, MD, an Oregon-based emergency medicine physician who has worked with the Himalayan Rescue Association. Information includes an explanation of altitude sickness, preventive measures, and treatments.

High Altitude Sickness
<http://familydoctor.org/handouts/247.html>

The handout featured on this site was created by the American Academy of Family Physicians to explain causes, prevention, and treatments for high altitude sickness.

ARTHRITIS

A Guide to Traveling with Arthritis
<http://www.marylandsorthopaedicteam.com/arthtrav.htm/>

The Orthopaedic Specialty Center in Baltimore, Maryland, offers tips for traveling with arthritis, including planning, traveling by air, traveling by automobile, and other information.

Living with Arthritis
<http://www.coxii.com/5_3_25.asp>

The Pharmacia Corporation manages the content on this site, also known as Arthritis.com. The information about automobile travel for arthritis sufferers covers the use of assistive devices (key holder, gas cap wrench) and requesting rental cars with helpful equipment (power windows, mirrors, brakes, and steering).

Travel and Arthritis
<http://www.arthritis.org/resources/travel/default.asp>

The Arthritis Foundation's information about travel and arthritis covers transportation (by plane, train, automobile), choosing destinations, and using arthritis-friendly automobiles.

☑ Traveling with Arthritis: Plan, Pack and Enjoy
<http://www.mayoclinic.com/invoke.cfm?id=HQ01554>

The Mayo Clinic advises travelers with arthritis to plan realistic trips, seek appropriate accommodations, pack light luggage, include extra medications, and consider the different modes of transportation, including airplane, train, bus, ship, and automobile.

BACK PROBLEMS

Back Pain on Vacation
<http://pptsonline.com/topics/topics_back_pain_vacation.htm>

Physicians Physical Therapy Service (PPTS) is an association of independent rehabilitation practices located in Arizona. The information about reducing back pain during vacation is practical and useful.

☑ **Back Pain Resource Center: Tips for Air Travel**
  <http://www.hopkinsafter50.com/html/silos/backpain/wpARTICLE_airtravel.php>

The Johns Hopkins University maintains a site titled Johns Hopkins Health After 50. This information about traveling by airplane with back pain covers precautions and in-flight exercise. The information is derived from a Johns Hopkins White Paper (authoritative report) about low back pain and osteoporosis. The page also includes information about traveling with medications.

Prevention: Traveling Back
  <http://www.backrelief.com/prevention/travel.html>

Whitehall-Robins is a Canadian pharmaceutical firm that sells medications to relieve back pain. Its traveling back information covers automobile travel, airplane travel, lodging, luggage, footwear, and tips for lifting heavy objects.

Top Tips for Travellers with Back Pain
  <http://www.backpain.org/pages/p_pages/pr-holiday.php>

The BackCare site is sponsored by the Charity for Healthier Backs, an organization that has the Prince of Wales as its patron. The site includes tips for travelers with back pain and sells information packs to the general public.

BITES AND STINGS

Bites and Stings
  <http://www.nlm.nih.gov/medlineplus/bitesandstings.html>

MedlinePlus organizes content and links about bites and stings, including general overviews, prevention and screening, specific conditions and aspects, treatment, organizations, and more.

Insect Precautions
<http://www.travelhealthline.com/z_insect.html>

Dr. Patrick Joseph is a travel medicine and infectious diseases practitioner who manages a travel clinic in San Francisco, California. His International Travel Healthline sells a report, but elsewhere on the site he offers freely accessible information about reducing the risk of insect bites and stings.

Insect Precautions
<http://www.cha.ab.ca/travellers/insects_animals.html>

This information about insect precautions is provided by Capital Health, a travel health service located in Edmonton, Alberta, Canada.

Marine-Life Stings and Bites
<http://www.healthsquare.com/mc/fgmc1413.htm>

HealthSquare information is provided by the publishers of *Physicians' Desk Reference*. Information includes signs and symptoms, wound care, and when to seek a physician's care.

☑ Protection Against Mosquitoes and Other Arthropods
<http://www.cdc.gov/travel/bugs.htm>

The U.S. Centers for Disease Control and Prevention (CDC) site covers vaccines, repellents, and general preventive measures used to avoid diseases transmitted by mosquitoes and other arthropods.

COLD WEATHER CONDITIONS

Arctic Health
<http://www.arctichealth.org/>

The U.S. National Library of Medicine (NLM) developed this portal devoted to Arctic health. Although it focuses primarily on the health issues of peoples native to the Arctic geographical area, some of the information may prove useful to persons traveling to the Arctic.

FEMA Factsheet: Winter Storms
\<http://www.fema.gov/hazards/winterstorms/stormsf.shtm\>

The Federal Emergency Management Association (FEMA) is an independent agency of the U.S. government that focuses on disaster prevention, preparedness, and recovery. The fact sheet about winter storms provides useful information about avoiding frostbite and other medical conditions associated with cold weather.

Frostbite
\<http://www.cdc.gov/nceh/hsb/extremecold/frostbite.htm\>

This overview of frostbite, developed by the U.S. Centers for Disease Control and Prevention (CDC), is of potential interest to travelers to cold climates.

Hypothermia and Cold Weather Injuries
\<http://www.princeton.edu/~oa/safety/hypocold.shtml\>

Written by Rick Curtis, who is associated with the Outdoor Action Program at Princeton University, this information on hypothermia and cold weather injuries is understandable, illustrated, and well referenced.

DEEP VEIN THROMBOSIS

Deep Vein Thrombosis and Air Travel
\<http://www.health.gov.au/pubhlth/strateg/communic/factsheets/thrombosis.htm\>

The Australian Department of Health and Ageing developed this site's fact sheet about deep vein thrombosis.

DVT Fact File
<http://www.aviation-health.org/dvtfacts.html>

The Aviation Health Institute, a nonprofit organization based in the United Kingdom, is dedicated to reducing health risks for persons who travel by air, especially deep vein thrombosis (DVT). The site features information about risk factors and methods of reducing risks.

Flight-Related Deep Vein Thrombosis
<http://ohp.nasa.gov//alerts/dvt.html>

The Occupational Health section of the National Aeronautics and Space Administration (NASA) site features useful information about the risk of deep vein thrombosis to aviators and passengers alike.

Spotlight Health's DVT
<http://www.spotlighthealth.com/dvt/dvt/dvt.htm>

Spotlight Health focuses on celebrity health stories. The information about deep vein thrombosis (DVT) describes the medical condition as experienced by Olympic figure skater Tara Lipinski, former Vice President Dan Quayle, Jethro Tull musician Ian Anderson, and former FBI profiler John Douglas. The celebrity anecdotes include images, video clips, and narrative paragraphs. The site also features information about support groups, DVT in the news, and resource links.

☑ Thrombophlebitis
<http://www.nlm.nih.gov/medlineplus/thrombophlebitis.html>

MedlinePlus organizes content and links about thrombophlebitis, including general overviews, clinical trials, diagnosis and symptoms, pictures and diagrams, prevention and screening, research, specific conditions and aspects, treatment, organizations, and more links related to the subject (see Figure 5.1).

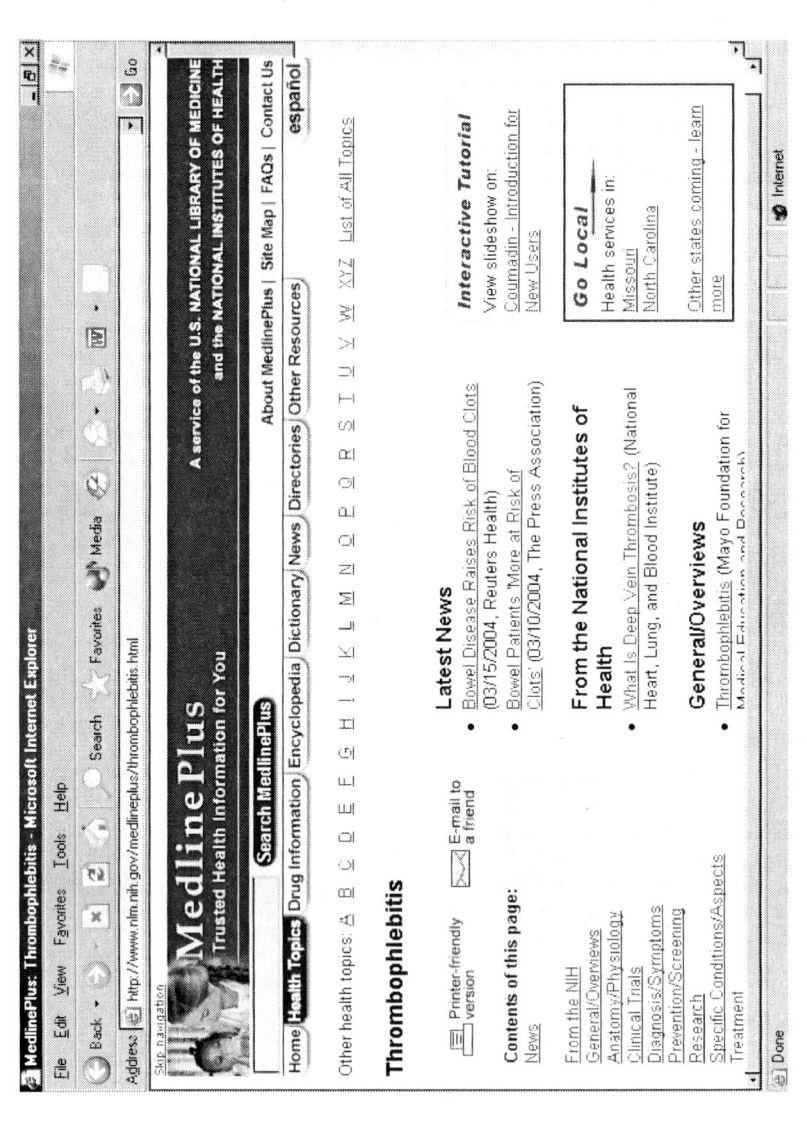

FIGURE 5.1. Thrombophlebitis, MedlinePlus Web Site

What's Behind "Economy Class Syndrome"?
<http://blueprint.bluecrossmn.com/topic/dvt;jsessionid=ZWNLMY3TJRZ52CTYAIUDF4Q>

On this page, BlueCross BlueShield of Minnesota describes economy class syndrome, or deep vein thrombosis, as a risk to inactive travelers on long flights.

DENGUE FEVER AND OTHER HEMORRHAGIC FEVERS

Dengue Fever
<http://www.travdoc.com/articles/art12.html>

TravDoc, a travel clinic located in Michigan, is the sponsor of this site, which discusses occurrence, symptoms, and treatment of dengue fever.

☑ Viral Hemorrhagic Fever
<http://www.cdc.gov/ncidod/diseases/virlfvr/virlfvr.htm>

The National Center for Infectious Diseases presents information about hemorrhagic fever (Ebola virus, Lassa fever, hantavirus), including fact sheets, risks and precautions for travelers, and blood-borne pathogens.

DENTAL PROBLEMS

☑ American Dental Association Directory
<http://www.ada.org/public/disclaimer.asp>

The American Dental Association (ADA) provides access to its directory of dentists, searchable by name, city, zip code, and specialty. This information is useful to persons traveling throughout the United States. Database results yield detailed maps to specific dental offices.

Dental Travel Kit
<http://www.dentalgentlecare.com/emergency%20travel%20kit.htm>

Dr. Dan Peterson of Family Gentle Dental Care in Gering, Nebraska, developed this useful list of supplies to equip a dental travel kit.

First Aid for Dental Emergencies
<http://www.healthy.net/LIBRARY/BOOKS/HEALTHY SELF/FIRSTAID/dental.htm>

This information about preventing and seeking first aid for dental emergencies was developed by the American Institute of Preventive Medicine.

International Dentists
<http://www.dental-resources.com/dentist3.html>

This site lists contact information for dentists located in countries from Australia to Uruguay. Another part of the site features dentists based in the United States.

DIABETES

International Diabetes Center: Travel
<http://www.parknicollet.com/diabetes/selfcare/travel.html>

The International Diabetes Center is located in Minneapolis, Minnesota. The site's travel information includes a travel checklist, planning tips, foot care advice, and advice on traveling overseas.

Travel to Developing Countries
<http://www.healthandage.com/Home/gm=6!gid6=105>

HealthandAge Network, a site maintained by the Novartis Foundation for Gerontology, develops content in cooperation with some major medical institutions. The information about traveling to developing countries was compiled by Massachusetts General Hospital and Harvard Medical School. The advice covers travelers with diabetes, travelers with heart and lung diseases, and pregnant travelers. The content on the site can be displayed in normal, large, and extralarge type sizes.

Traveling with Diabetes
<http://www.warrenclinic.com/services/diabetes/traveling.asp>

The Warren Clinic is part of the St. Francis Health System in Tulsa, Oklahoma. This site's information about traveling with diabetes covers advance planning, a packing checklist, and insulin adjustments.

☑ Traveling with Diabetes Supplies
<http://www.diabetes.org/advocacy-and-legalresources/discrimination/public_accommodation/travel.jsp>

The American Diabetes Association provides advice for persons with diabetes traveling with insulin and syringes in light of recently heightened airport security.

☑ When You Travel
<http://www.diabetes.org/main/type-1-diabetes/travel.jsp>

The American Diabetes Association's site offers sound advice for healthy travel for persons with diabetes.

DIARRHEA

☑ Amebiasis: Health Information for International Travel
<http://www.cdc.gov/travel/diseases/amebiasis.htm>

The National Center for Infectious Diseases, part of the U.S. Centers for Disease Control and Prevention (CDC), provides information about amebiasis, caused by microscopic parasites, which can cause diarrheal and liver diseases. Information includes a brief description, risk for travelers, preventive measures, and treatment.

☑ Diarrhea
<http://www.nlm.nih.gov/medlineplus/diarrhea.html>

MedlinePlus organizes content and links about diarrhea, including general overviews, clinical trials, diagnosis and symptoms, pictures and diagrams, research, specific conditions and aspects, dictionaries and glossaries, organizations, and more.

☑ Travelers' Diarrhea
<http://www.cdc.gov/ncidod/dbmd/diseaseinfo/travelers diarrhea_g.htm>

The Division of Bacterial and Mycotic Diseases of the U.S. Centers for Disease Control and Prevention (CDC) provides general information about the causes, preventive measures, and treatment of diarrhea developed by travelers.

EAR PROBLEMS

☑ Ears and Altitude
<http://www.entnet.org/healthinfo/ears/altitude.cfm>

The American Academy of Otolaryngology—Head and Neck Surgery developed this page's content about the effects of air travel on the ear.

Travel Tips for Hearing Impaired People
<http://www.janela1.com/vh/docs/v0001339.htm>

The American Academy of Otolaryngology—Head and Neck Surgery describes the difficulties and challenges experienced by hearing impaired travelers. The page lists major airlines that use TDD (telecommunication device for the deaf) equipment to communicate with customers.

EXERCISE BEFORE AND DURING TRAVEL

On-the-Road Fitness Resources
<http://www.zyworld.com/MFedin/WC2CFitness.htm>

The Wellness Concierge presents information on packable exercise equipment, yoga to go, locating health clubs while traveling, and other useful content.

Stretching for Travelers
<http://www.ricksteves.com/news/0106/stretch.htm>

The travel site maintained by travel writer Rick Steves includes stretching tips for travelers.

Travel Exercise and Diet Guidelines
<http://www.travelfitness.com/>

The Travel Fitness site features tips and suggestions based on the book *Travel Fitness: Feel Better, Perform Better on the Road,* written by Rebecca Johnson and Bill Tulin. Features include pretravel conditioning exercises, packing lists, and a workout quiz.

Travel Fitness
<http://carlisle-www.army.mil/apfri/travel_fitness.htm>

The Army Physical Fitness Research Institute (APFRI) is located at the U.S. Army War College at Carlisle Barracks, Pennsylvania. APFRI's site features travel fitness tips, including maintaining aerobic fitness while traveling and the effects of travel on aerobic capacity.

Traveling: Fitness on the Road
<http://www.ivillage.com/diet/experts/fitfriday/articles/0,5050,253455_93363-2,00.html>

iVillage is a commercial site that serves as an online community for women. The information about fitness on the road includes a no-equipment workout that can be done anywhere, including in hotels, on airplanes, and in automobiles.

Workouts That Travel
<http://www.workoutsforyou.com/article_travel.htm>

Workouts For You is a commercial site that markets customized workouts. The travel workouts are simple and practical.

FEAR OF FLYING

Anxiety Coach: Overcoming the Fear of Flying
<http://www.anxietycoach.com/flying.htm>

Anxietycoach.com is a site that includes advice from Dr. David A. Carbonell, a clinical psychologist. The information about fear of flying focuses on causes and treatments.

Fear of Flying Clinic
<http://www.fofc.com/>

The Fear of Flying Clinic is located at the San Francisco International Airport in San Mateo, California. The site includes frequently asked questions, a list of scheduled classes, and a message board.

Fear of Flying Information Sources
<http://www.airsafe.com/issues/fear.htm>

The AirSafe.com site includes a selection of information sources about fear of flying.

SOAR
<http://www.fearofflying.com/>

SOAR is an organization that helps people address their fear of flying through instructional materials, counseling, workshops, chat sessions, and message board discussions.

FOOD-BORNE ILLNESSES

☑ Food Contamination and Poisoning
<http://www.nlm.nih.gov/medlineplus/foodcontamination poisoning.html>

MedlinePlus organizes content and links, including the latest news about food-borne illnesses, as well as general overviews, clinical trials, diagnosis and symptoms, pictures and diagrams, prevention and screening, specific conditions and aspects, organizations, content in other languages, and more.

☑ Food Safety While Hiking, Camping, and Boating
<http://www.fsis.usda.gov/OA/pubs/hcb.htm>

The Food Safety and Inspection Service of the U.S. Department of Agriculture (USDA) explains methods of keeping food and water safe to consume while hiking, camping, and boating.

☑ Foodborne Diseases
<http://www.niaid.nih.gov/factsheets/foodbornedis.htm>

The National Institute of Allergy and Infectious Diseases of the U.S. National Institutes of Health (NIH) developed this fact sheet related to typical food-borne illnesses, including botulism, campylobacteriosis, *E. coli* infections, salmonellosis, shigellosis, etc.

Organisms That Can Bug You
<http://www.fightbac.org/bug.cfm>

The Partnership for Food Safety Education is a U.S.-based public-private partnership that strives to educate the public about safe food-handling practices. The site includes a chart of organisms, sources of illness, and symptoms.

☑ **Risks from Food and Drink**
<http://www.cdc.gov/travel/food-drink-risks.htm>

The Travelers' Health site maintained by the National Center for Infectious Diseases of the U.S. Centers for Disease Control and Prevention (CDC) includes information about risks from food and drink, along with methods of treating water to make it safe to drink.

HEPATITIS

☑ **Hepatitis**
<http://www.nlm.nih.gov/medlineplus/hepatitis.html>

MedlinePlus organizes content and links including the latest news about hepatitis, as well as general overviews, clinical trials, diagnosis and symptoms, disease management, prevention and screening, specific conditions and aspects, organizations, statistics, and more.

☑ **Hepatitis A and B: Health Information for International Travel**
<http://www.cdc.gov/travel/diseases/hav.htm> and
<http://www.cdc.gov/travel/diseases/hbv.htm>

The National Center for Infectious Diseases maintains travel health content on the U.S. Centers for Disease Control and Prevention (CDC) site. The information about Hepatitis A and B includes an understandable disease description, occurrence, risk for travelers, preventive measures, and links to other information.

☑ **Viral Hepatitis A through E and Beyond**
<http://www.niddk.nih.gov/health/digest/pubs/hep/hepa-e/hepa-e.htm>

The National Institute of Diabetes and Digestive and Kidney Diseases (NIDDK), part of the U.S. National Institutes of Health (NIH), details on its site the disease spread, people at risk, prevention, and treatment for hepatitis A, B, C, D, and E, which are diseases of risk to travelers.

HIV AND AIDS

☑ CDC Travelers' Health Information on AIDS
<http://www.cdc.gov/travel/diseases/hivaids.htm> and <http://www.cdc.gov/travel/hivtrav.htm>

The National Center for Infectious Diseases maintains content about occurrence, risk to travelers, and prevention of HIV and AIDS on the U.S. Centers for Disease Control and Prevention (CDC) site, especially as it relates to travel.

☑ HIV Testing Requirements
<http://travel.state.gov/HIVtestingreqs.html>

The U.S. State Department site lists country-specific requirements for HIV test results needed for travelers planning extended stays in foreign countries.

Immunizations for Immunocompromised Travelers
<http://www.mdtravelhealth.com/special/Immunocompromised.html>

Intended for travelers and physicians alike, this site describes itself as "a limited liability corporation based in Scarsdale, N.Y.," with the content developed by David Goldberg, MD, a member of the International Society of Travel Medicine and the American Society of Tropical Medicine and Hygiene. The recommendations for immunocompromised travelers cover avoiding vaccinations with live viruses and taking precautions with foods and beverages. The site also includes useful external links.

JET LAG

How to Beat Jetlag
<http://www.alltraveltips.com/beatjetlag.shtml>

AllTravelTips.com is a commercial site that includes useful information for travelers, including how to minimize the effects of jet lag.

Jet Lag
<http://blueprint.bluecrossmn.com/topic/jetlag;jsessionid=ZWNLMY3TJRZ52CTYAIUDF4Q>

BlueCross BlueShield of Minnesota offers detailed advice for minimizing the effects of jet lag. The content comes from Consumer Health Interactive (http://www.consumerhi.com/), whose content is reviewed by physicians.

Jetlag—Sleepchannel
<http://www.sleepdisorderchannel.net/jetlag/>

The Sleepchannel features content written by physicians specializing in sleep disorders; pulmonary medicine; and ear, nose, and throat diseases. The information about jet lag covers symptoms, causes, and management. Circadian rhythms are also discussed.

Jet-Lag: Symptoms and Treatment
<http://www.sportsci.org/encyc/jetlag/jetlag.html>

This site includes an *Encyclopedia of Sports Medicine and Science* chapter on jet lag, written by Thomas Reilly of Liverpool John Moores University in England.

☑ Sleep and the Traveler
<http:/www.sleepfoundation.org/publications/travel.html>

The Sleep Foundation is a nonprofit organization that supports education and research related to sleep and sleep disorders. Content on this site of interest to travelers includes tips for getting sufficient rest before, during, and after travel, and how to reduce the harmful effects of jet lag.

Slumber Strategies for the Sleep-Deprived
<http://www.zyworld.com/MFedin/WC2SleepMain.htm>

The Wellness Concierge site presents information about power-sleep basics, sleep aids, environmental factors, and links to external sites.

Techniques for Reducing Jet Lag
<http://www.nojetlag.com/jetlag3.html>

Nojetlag.com is a site that sells homeopathic products to treat jet lag. The site also include techniques for reducing the effects of jet lag without any medications.

LUNG DISEASES

☑ Air Travel for Patients with TB
<http://www.dhs.vic.gov.au/phd/tb/airtravel.htm>

Australia's Victorian Government Health Information on air travel by persons with tuberculosis (TB) covers the risk of transmission to others, continuation of therapy, recommended reading, and more.

☑ SARS
<http://www.emerginginfections.slu.edu/sars.htm>

The Center for the Study of Emerging Infections is located at the St. Louis University School of Public Health. The site's information about SARS includes fact sheets, reports, training, news, key references, and links to other public health information about SARS.

☑ **SARS Information for Travelers**
<http://www.cdc.gov/ncidod/sars/qa/travel.htm>

The National Center for Infectious Diseases maintains travel health content on the U.S. Centers for Disease Control and Prevention (CDC) site. The information about severe acute respiratory syndrome (SARS) includes travel restrictions, precautions, and infection control practices.

☑ **SARS Update**
<http://www.cmaj.ca/misc/sars.shtml>

The *Canadian Medical Association Journal (CMAJ)* consolidates information from the World Health Organization (WHO), the U.S. Centers for Disease Control and Prevention (CDC), and Health Canada to provide case definition, management of cases, and prevention and control information about SARS.

☑ **Severe Acute Respiratory Syndrome**
<http://www.nlm.nih.gov/medlineplus/severeacute respiratorysyndrome.html>

MedlinePlus organizes content and links, including the latest news about SARS, as well as general overviews, clinical trials, diagnosis and symptoms, pictures and diagrams, specific conditions and aspects, organizations, and more.

☑ **Severe Acute Respiratory Syndrome (SARS) and Coronavirus Testing**
<http://www.cdc.gov/mmwr/preview/mmwrhtml/ mm5214a1.htm>

This information about SARS was published originally in the Centers for Disease Control and Prevention's (CDC) *Morbidity and Mortality Weekly Review.*

☑ **Summary of SARS and Air Travel**
<http://www.who.int/csr/sars/travel/airtravel/en>

The World Health Organization (WHO) details the risk of SARS transmission during an airline flight, in-flight precautions, and the disinfection of aircraft (see Figure 5.2).

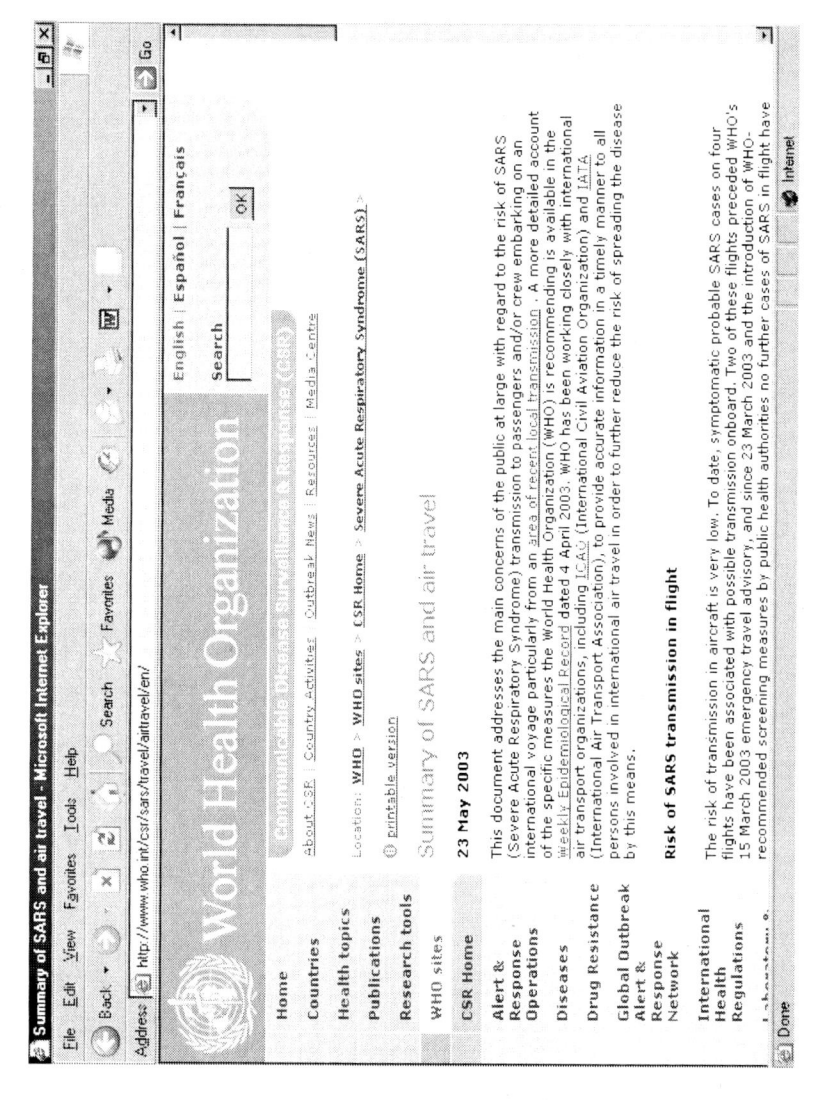

FIGURE 5.2. Summary of SARS and Air Travel, World Health Organization (WHO) Web Site

Travel to Developing Countries
   <http://www.healthandage.com/Home/gm=6!gid6=105>

HealthandAge Network, a site maintained by the Novartis Foundation for Gerontology, provides content developed in cooperation with some major medical institutions. The information about traveling to developing countries was developed by Massachusetts General Hospital and Harvard Medical School. The advice covers travelers with diabetes or heart and lung diseases as well as pregnant travelers. The content on the site can be displayed in normal, large, and extra large type sizes.

☑ **Tuberculosis**
   <http://www.umm.edu/travel/tuberc.htm>

The Travel Medicine site developed by University of Maryland Medicine describes tuberculosis, including the risk of developing the disease, symptoms, etiology, diagnosis, and treatment. The page's content can be translated into German, Spanish, Portuguese, French, or Italian by clicking a box.

LYME DISEASE

☑ **Lyme Disease**
   <http://www.nlm.nih.gov/medlineplus/lymedisease.html>

MedlinePlus organizes content and links, including the latest news about lyme disease, as well as general overviews, clinical trials, diagnosis and symptoms, pictures and diagrams, specific conditions and aspects, organizations, and more.

Lyme Disease
   <http://kidshealth.org/teen/infections/skin_rashes/lyme_
   disease.html>

KidsHealth is funded by the Nemours Foundation, an organization dedicated to improving children's health. The information about lyme disease is understandable, illustrated, and useful for children living in or traveling to infested areas.

☑ We Want You to Know About Lyme Disease: It's Difficult to Diagnose
<http://www.fda.gov/cdrh/consumer/lymedisease.html>

The U.S. Food and Drug Administration (FDA) site provides information about lyme disease, including transmission, symptoms, diagnosis, treatment, and precautions.

MAD COW DISEASE

☑ Bovine Spongiform Encephalopathy
<http://www.fda.gov/oc/opacom/hottopics/bse.html>

The U.S. Food and Drug Administration (FDA) has organized information related to bovine spongiform encephalopathy (mad cow disease), including general background, recent actions, consumer information, industry and veterinary information, bovine-based vaccines, and blood safety.

☑ Bovine Spongiform Encephalopathy and Variant Creutzfeldt-Jakob Disease
<http://www.cdc.gov/travel/diseases/madcow.htm>

The U.S. Centers for Disease Control and Prevention (CDC) developed this information on bovine spongiform encephalopathy (mad cow disease), including a disease description as well as data on its occurrence, the risk for travelers, and prevention.

MALARIA

☑ Malaria
<http://www.nlm.nih.gov/medlineplus/malaria.html>

MedlinePlus organizes content and links about malaria, including general overviews, clinical trials, prevention and screening, research, specific conditions and aspects, treatment, organizations, and more.

☑ Malaria: How to Prevent It
<http:/familydoctor.org/handouts/384.html>

FamilyDoctor is a site developed by the American Academy of Family Physicians. The information about malaria covers prevention, treatment, and links to more information.

☑ Malaria Prophylaxis
<http://ohp.nasa.gov/topics/traveler/malaria.html>

The Occupational Health section of the National Aeronautics and Space Administration (NASA) site features useful information about the risk of malaria to aviators and passengers alike.

☑ Regional Malaria Information
<http://www.cdc.gov/travel/regionalmalaria>

The National Center for Infectious Diseases maintains travel health content on the U.S. Centers for Disease Control and Prevention (CDC) site. The information about malaria includes an understandable disease description, occurrence, risk for travelers, preventive measures, and links to other information.

MOTION SICKNESS

MD Travel Health—Motion Sickness
<http://www.mdtravelhealth.com/illness/motion_sickness.html>

MD Travel Health's content is maintained and updated by David Goldberg, MD, a physician with training in internal medicine and infectious diseases. The content about motion sickness covers treatment and techniques for reducing symptoms.

☑ Motion Sickness
<http://www.nlm.nih.gov/medlineplus/motionsickness.html>

MedlinePlus organizes content and links about motion sickness, including general overviews, anatomy and physiology, organizations, how the ailment affects children, and more.

PREGNANCY

☑ Air Travel During Pregnancy
<http://www.acog.org/from_home/publications/press_releases/nr12-12-01-3.cfm>

The American College of Obstetricians and Gynecologists (ACOG) addressed the risks of air travel during pregnancy in this press release from 2001.

Airline Policies for Pregnant Travelers
<http://www.babycenter.com/general/pregnancytravel/pregnancy/6976.html>

BabyCenter is a commercial site with information about preconception, pregnancy, babies, toddlers, and other subjects. The section about pregnant travelers includes concise airline policy information with links and toll-free numbers.

Eight Smart Strategies for Pregnant Travelers
<http://www.babycenter.com/refcap/pregnancy/pregnancytravel/6977.html>

BabyCenter's smart strategies for pregnant travelers section includes information about reducing stress, staying comfortable, eating and drinking, avoiding yeast infections, and more.

☑ **Guidelines for Vaccinating Pregnant Women**
  <http://www.cdc.gov/nip/publications/preg_guide.htm>

Although the National Immunization Program section of the U.S. Centers for Disease Control and Prevention (CDC) emphasizes routine child and adult immunization schedules, the site also includes useful information for pregnant women planning to travel to areas that require additional immunizations. The fifteen-page guide was updated in October 2003.

☑ **International Travel and Health: Pregnancy**
  <http://www.who.int/ith/chapter06_16.html#pregnancy>

The World Health Organization (WHO) publishes *International Travel and Health,* which includes a chart of vaccines both recommended and not recommended for pregnant women.

Pregnancy
  <http://www.aviation-health.org/pregnancy.html>

The Aviation Health Institute provides brief information about air travel during pregnancy.

☑ **Pregnancy, Breast-Feeding, and Travel**
  <http://www.cdc.gov/travel/pregnant.htm>

The National Center for Infectious Diseases maintains travel health content on the U.S. Centers for Disease Control and Prevention (CDC) site. The information about pregnancy and breast-feeding includes factors that can affect decisions to travel, contraindications to international travel, recommended immunizations/vaccinations, information on malaria and diarrhea, and a recommended travel health kit for pregnant travelers.

Travel to Developing Countries
  <http://www.healthandage.com/Home/gm=6!gid6=105>

HealthandAge Network, a site maintained by the Novartis Foundation for Gerontology, provides content developed in cooperation with some major medical institutions. The information about traveling to developing countries was developed by Massachusetts General Hospital and Harvard Medical School. The advice covers pregnant travelers, as well as travelers with diabetes and heart and lung diseases. The content on the site can be displayed in normal, large, and extra large type sizes.

Travelling During Pregnancy
<http://www.babyworld.co.uk/information/pregnancy/travel/travel.asp>

Based in the United Kingdom, Radcliffe Medical Press launched babyworld.co.uk as a portal of information for present and future parents. The content about traveling during pregnancy includes a discussion board, trip-planning advice, emergency medical supplies, and other information.

SUNBURN, SUNSTROKE, AND HEAT EXHAUSTION

☑ Choose Your Cover
<http://www.cdc.gov/ChooseYourCover/qanda.htm>

The U.S. Centers for Disease Control and Prevention (CDC) site includes information from the National Center for Chronic Disease Prevention and Health Promotion about skin cancer prevention. The information includes questions and answers about sun exposure, sunburn, ultraviolet rays, and protective clothing.

☑ FEMA—Fact Sheet: Extreme Heat
<http://www.fema.gov/hazards/extremeheat/heatf.shtm>

The Federal Emergency Management Agency (FEMA) of the U.S. government developed this fact sheet to explain the risks of extreme heat, including the symptoms of heat disorders (sunburn, sunstroke, heat exhaustion), and basic first aid advice for treating conditions resulting from extreme heat.

Heat Cramps, Heat Exhaustion, and Heat Stroke
<http://www.drreddy.com/heat.html>

Dr. Vinay Reddy is a pediatrician who practices medicine in Kalamazoo, Michigan, and teaches pediatric residents at Michigan State University. Site information covers symptoms and preventive measures for heat cramps, heat exhaustion, and heat stroke.

How to Avoid Becoming a Heat Casualty
<http://www.zyworld.com/MFedin/RR/April18.htm>

The Wellness Concierge includes health advice from Dr. Stuart Rose and other experts about avoiding illnesses associated with heat exposure, including staying hydrated, avoiding diuretics, and recognizing the symptoms of heat exhaustion.

☑ Sun Exposure
<http://www.nlm.nih.gov/medlineplus/sunexposure.html>

MedlinePlus organizes content and links, including the latest news about sun exposure as well as general overviews, clinical trials, diagnosis and symptoms, pictures and diagrams, specific conditions and aspects, organizations, and more.

Sun Exposure
<http://www.thetraveldoctor.com/sun.html>

Travel Medicine Consultants, based in Dallas, Texas, maintains this site, which includes medical advice from internal medicine physicians Dr. Mark A. Johnston and Dr. Paul Sanders. The information about sunstroke includes tips on sunscreens, ultraviolet light, and sunglasses.

Sun Safety
<http://kidshealth.org/parent/firstaid_safe/outdoor/sun_safety.html>

KidsHealth is funded by the Nemours Foundation, an organization dedicated to improving children's health. The information about sun safety covers the dangers of ultraviolet (UV) radiation; using protective clothing, sunscreen, and eyewear; and treating sunburned skin.

WEST NILE VIRUS

☑ CDC West Nile Virus Home Page
<http://www.cdc.gov/ncidod/dvbid/westnile/2002spotlight.htm>

The Division of Vector-Borne Infectious Diseases, part of the U.S. Centers for Disease Control and Prevention (CDC), offers three approaches for reducing the risk of West Nile virus: avoiding mosquito bites, mosquito-proofing the home, and working with the community to eliminate conditions that increase disease transmission. The site also includes maps of West Nile virus activity in the United States.

Disease Information: West Nile Virus
<http://www.hc-sc.gc.ca/pphb-dgspsp/tmp-pmv/info/wnv_e.html>

The Health Canada site provides a disease profile of West Nile virus, including disease transmission, geographic distribution, symptoms, risk, and prevention.

☑ MedlinePlus: West Nile Virus
<http://www.nlm.nih.gov/medlineplus/westnilevirus.html>

MedlinePlus organizes content and links about West Nile virus, including the latest news, general overviews, diagnosis and symptoms, pictures and diagrams, prevention and screening, specific conditions and aspects, treatment, statistics, and more.

West Nile Virus
<http://www.travelhealth.co.uk/diseases/westnile.htm>

TravelHealth.co.uk has partnered with the United Kingdom's Foreign and Commonwealth Office (FCO) to provide information needed for British travelers to remain safe and healthy. The information about West Nile virus covers risks and tips for prevention.

YELLOW FEVER

☑ **Yellow Fever**
<http://www.umm.edu/travel/yellow.htm>

The University of Maryland Medicine site features information related to travel medicine. The brief information about yellow fever describes transmission, symptoms, prevention, and treatment. Content can be translated into German, Spanish, Portuguese, French, or Italian by clicking a box.

Yellow Fever
<http://www.astdhpphe.org/infect/yellow.html>

The Association of State and Territorial Directors of Health Promotion and Public Health Education (ASTDHPPHE) has organized information about a variety of infectious diseases, including yellow fever. The yellow fever facts include likely places to contract the disease, transmission, symptoms, diagnosis, treatment, and prevention.

☑ **Yellow Fever, 2002**
<http://www.who.int/ith/chapter05_m12_yellowf.html>

The World Health Organization (WHO) information about yellow fever includes a world map depicting areas of South America and Africa where the disease is endemic and a checklist for travelers (see Figure 5.3).

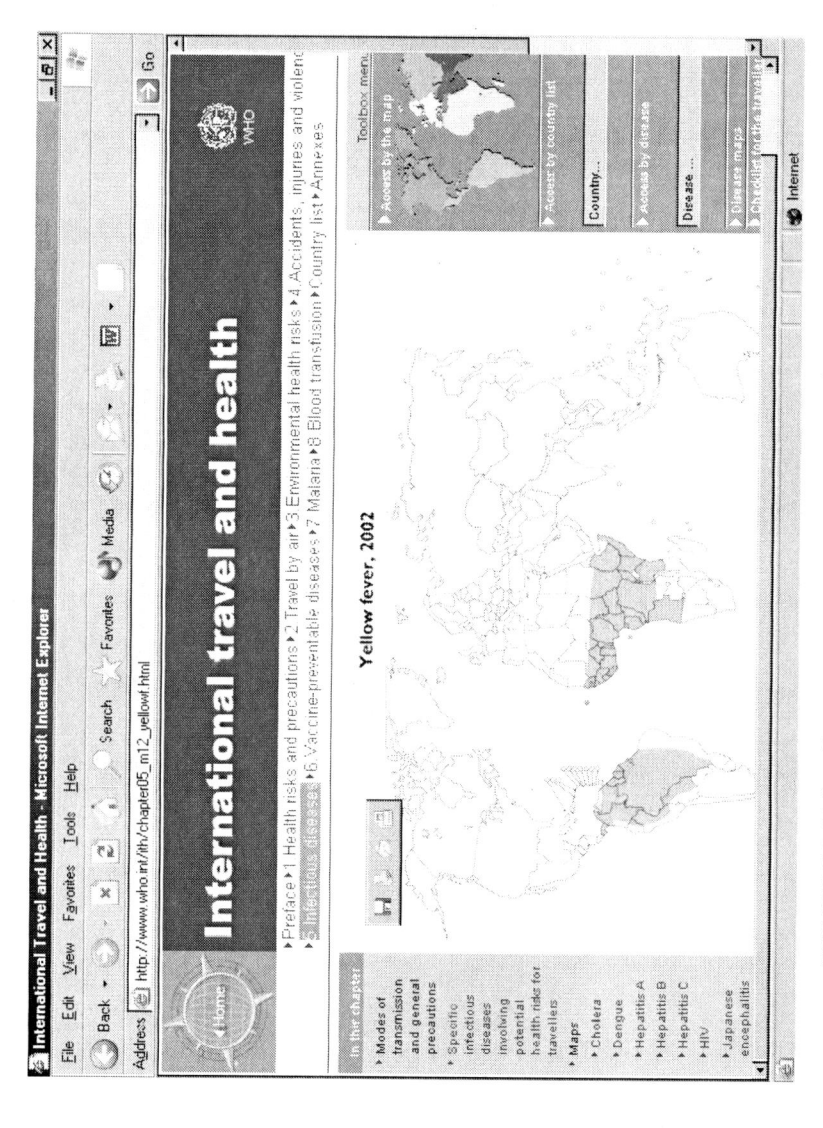

FIGURE 5.3. Yellow Fever, 2002, World Health Organization (WHO) Web Site

Chapter 6

Interactive Tools

Some Web sites feature tools that generate dynamic content based on input from site visitors. For example, driving distance calculators use starting and end points to calculate the traveling time and mileage between two locations. Other sites dispense real-time travel advice, including traffic congestion reports, weather conditions, and crash statistics. This chapter includes interactive tools of use to travelers or persons planning to travel.

AAA Foundation for Traffic Safety
<http://www.aaafoundation.org/resources/>

The AAA Foundation for Traffic Safety works to prevent traffic crashes through educational outreach and research. The site includes online quizzes and educational materials about distracted driving, child safety seats, drowsy driving, and other topics.

AccuWeather
<http://www.accuweather.com/adcbin/public/int_maps_menu.asp?nav=int>

The AccuWeather site includes an interactive section that accesses daily and extended forecast maps for specific geographical regions of the world (see Figure 6.1). The forecasts cover precipitation, ultraviolet (UV) index, winds, and high and low temperatures.

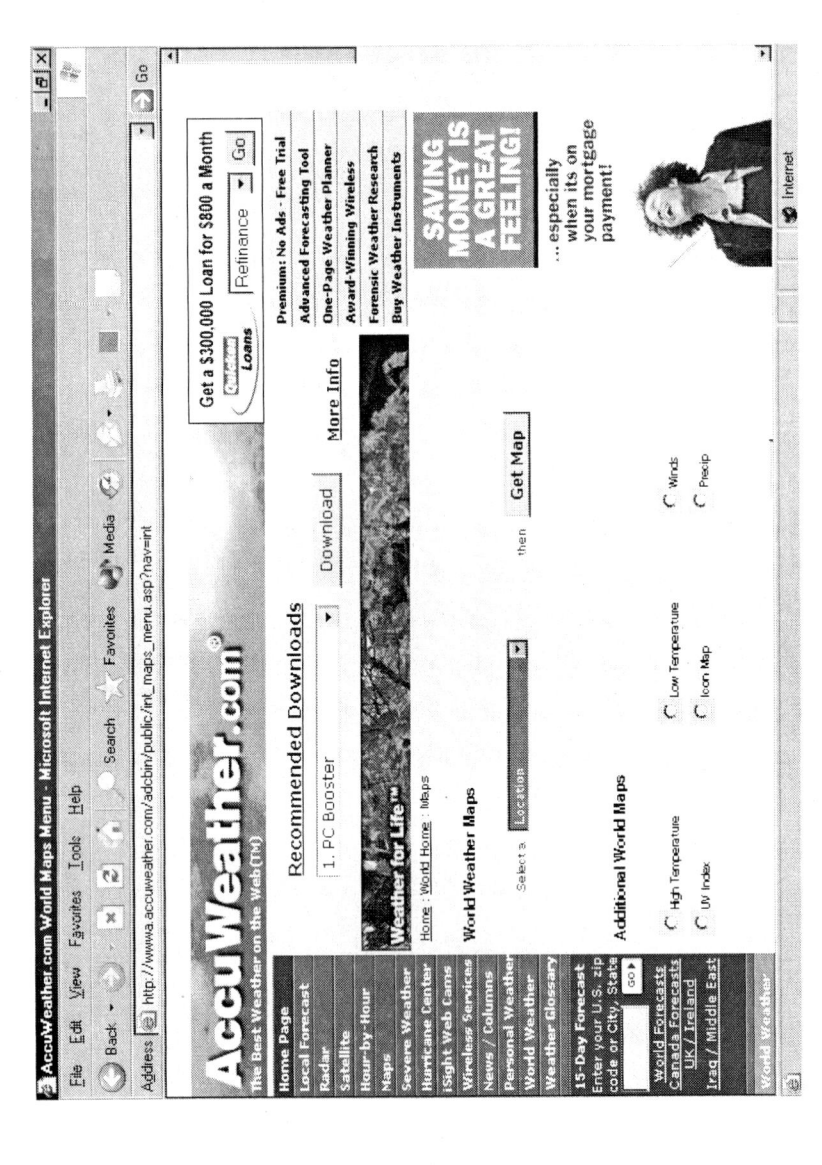

FIGURE 6.1. World Weather Maps, AccuWeather Web Site

Air Quality Forecast
<http://www.weather.com/activities/health/airquality/?par =Desktop>

The Weather Channel site includes air quality forecasts and maps searchable by U.S. state.

Air Traffic Control System Command Center
<http://www.fly.faa.gov/flyfaa/usmap.jsp>

The U.S. Federal Aviation Administration's Air Traffic Control System Command Center provides real-time status on air flight arrival and departure delays.

Aircraft Crashes Records Office
<http://www.baaa-acro.com/>

The Aircraft Crashes Records Office (Bureau d'Archives des Accidents Aéronautiques) is located in Geneva, Switzerland. The site features a searchable database of accident news and statistics dating back as far as 1919, and photographs dating back to 1930. Information about specific air crashes includes date of crash, type of aircraft, airline company, and accident site.

Ask the Doctor
<http://www.netdoctor.co.uk/q_a/index.asp>

Netdoctor.co.uk is a British site that features a team of general practitioners available to answer questions twenty-four hours a day, seven days a week. The site warns that not every question can be answered but does ensure that e-mail acknowledgments are sent to inquirers within four days. The site also includes the answers to the latest questions posted by other site visitors.

Combined Health Information Database (CHID)
<http://chid.nih.gov/>

CHID is a bibliographic database that combines the consumer health efforts of various U.S. government agencies. Typical search results yield bibliographic citations to consumer health publications available from a variety of sources.

Destinations
<http://www.cdc.gov/travel/destinat.htm>

The National Center for Infectious Diseases of the U.S. Centers for Disease Control and Prevention (CDC) developed this interactive world map to present information about diseases and disease risks in specific geographic regions.

Drivers.com
<http://www.drivers.com/>

PDE Publications, Inc., specializes in information about driving and driving behavior. This site includes news, discussions, and traffic safety information.

Driving Tests
<http://www.drdriving.org/surveys/#Tests>

The Drdriving site has organized a list of links to various aggressive driving tests.

Healthy Travel Quiz
<http://www.prevention.com/cda/quizleadin2002/1,4772,573,00.html>

Rodale, Inc., publisher of *Prevention* magazine and other consumer health information, developed this companion site that focuses on the same subjects. This brief quiz is intended to promote healthy travel habits.

Jet Lag Calculator
<http://www.masta.org/travel-tools/jetcalc.asp>

MASTA's jet lag calculator prompts the entry of travel details (starting place, ending place, direction, length of stay, and normal sleep times) in order to provide individualized feedback. An American living on the East Coast and traveling to France, for example, would discover that the trip spans five time zones and that he or she should drink sufficient nonalcoholic fluids to prevent dehydration during the flight, as well as get plenty of rest and exposure to light upon reaching the destination, to minimize the effects of jet lag.

MapQuest
<http://www.mapquest.com/>

Although not related to travel health, this site is useful for calculating travel distances, getting driving directions, creating maps, and developing travel plans for locations in the United States.

National Traffic and Road Closure Information
<http://www.fhwa.dot.gov/trafficinfo/index.htm>

The Federal Highway Administration of the U.S. Department of Transportation (DOT) site provides information about road closures, traffic warnings, traffic cameras, road construction, road conditions, weather, and more, organized by state.

Project ACTION Accessible Traveler's Database
<http://projectaction.easterseals.com/site/PageServer?pagename=ESPA_homepage>

The Project ACTION Accessible Traveler's Database provides information about public transit operators, accessible van rental companies, private bus and tour companies with accessible vehicles, accessible taxicabs, accessible airport transportation at selected airports, and more. The database is searchable by state and city.

Quiz—Do You Know How to Travel Safely?
<http://blueprint.bluecrossmn.com/topic/safetravelquiz;jsessionid=ZWNLMY3TJRZ52CTYAIUDF4Q>

BlueCross BlueShield of Minnesota developed this quiz to assess knowledge of jet lag, motion sickness, getting sick abroad, and other topics.

Real Time Traffic Congestion Maps
<http://traffic.tann.net/>

The Travel Advisory News Network (TANN) site covers traffic tips, travel alerts, and real-time traffic congestion maps for selected cities in Arizona, California, New York, Texas, and other states.

SmarTraveler
<http://www.smartraveler.com/>

This site's traffic reports are route specific and generate real-time data for traffic conditions in Boston, south Florida, and the Philadelphia area.

Temperature Converter
<http://www.world-travel-net.com/wtn/tools/temperature.asp>

This temperature tool can be used to convert temperatures from Fahrenheit to Centigrade and Centigrade to Fahrenheit. The site also features the tool as a small pop-up window.

Temperature Forecast Map
<http://www.usatoday.com/weather/forecast/wglobe.htm>

The USAToday.com site features an interactive world map that shows high temperature forecasts and weather conditions for major cities in major geographic areas.

Traffic Reports
<http://www.traffic.com/>

Traffic.com is a site maintained by Mobility Technologies, a company that develops traffic network information for television, radio, and cable networks. The traffic reports on this site are organized by U.S. city, from Baltimore to Tampa. The real-time data include a metropolitan map of incidents, alerts, advisories, and events that can affect traffic flow.

TRAVAX
<http://www.travax.scot.nhs.uk/InfoPage.htm>

The Travel Health Division of the Scottish Centre for Infection and Environmental Health (SCIEH) maintains and updates TRAVAX, an interactive database with current travel health information for health professionals. Database information "reflects the consensus views of the TRAVAX Advisory Panel made up of medical and nursing experts from different specialties."

Travel Clinic Directory
<http://www.astmh.org/scripts/clinindex.asp>

The American Society of Tropical Medicine and Hygiene (ASTMH) provides a database of travel clinics located throughout the world, searchable by country or state/province. Typical entries include name of physician, phone and fax numbers, e-mail address, Web site address, hours available, and description of clinic services. The physician directory lists members of ASTMH.

Travel Health Advisory Report
<http://www.tmvc.com.au/travelreport.asp?UnqID= 0.1421748andPageID=10>

Travel Doctor (TVMC), with travel clinics in Australia and New Zealand, provides a dynamic feature that generates a health advisory report for specific destinations. The reports feature country-specific information about immunizations, potential exposure to infectious diseases, Department of Foreign Affairs travel advice, embassy information, etc.

Weather Window
<http://www.cnn.com/WEATHER/>

CNN's weather information and forecasts can be customized by U.S. zip code or city name.

Chapter 7

Organizations

Various professional and civic organizations throughout the world focus on issues of concern to travelers. Many of these organizations publish pamphlets, journals, and reports useful to persons planning to travel. The ☑ symbol is used to denote organizational sites of major significance to travelers.

American Society of Travel Agents (ASTA)
<http://www.astanet.com/>

ASTAnet is the network site of the American Society of Travel Agents. Site features include travel headlines, alerts, health and safety tips, and more.

☑ American Society of Tropical Medicine and Hygiene (ASTMH)
<http://www.astmh.org/>

ASTMH focuses on the prevention and treatment of parasitic and viral diseases of the tropics, enteric infectious diseases, and mycobacterial infectious diseases. The site provides a travel clinic directory and links to publications, including the *American Journal of Tropical Medicine and Hygiene* and *Tropical Medicine and Hygiene News*.

Association for Safe International Road Travel (ASIRT)
<http://www.asirt.org/>

ASIRT was founded in 1995 after a young American citizen was killed in a bus crash in Turkey that killed twenty-one other passengers. Site features include Tourism and Travel, Travel Toolbox, Road Travel Reports, Global Safety, Publications, Links, Seasonal Hazards, and other information.

Association of State and Territorial Health Officials (ASTHO)
<http://www.astho.org/>

ASTHO "is the national nonprofit organization representing the state and territorial public health agencies of the United States, the U.S. Territories, and the District of Columbia." The ASTHO site includes information about organizational activities, programs, public health advocacy, events, and policy statements.

British Travel Health Association (BTHA)
<http://www.btha.org/>

BTHA strives to "promote a multi-disciplinary approach to travel health; provide a forum for discussion and information exchange; offer information and education; promote research on travel health issues; [and] increase public awareness of travel health hazards." Features include news, past copies of its Travel Wise newsletter, and travel health links.

☑ Canadian Society for International Health (CSIH)
<http://www.csih.org/trav_inf.html>

CSIH is a Canadian-based nongovernmental organization dedicated to international health and development. Site features include links to Canadian embassies and missions abroad, travel information and advisory reports, and other information.

☑ Centers for Disease Control and Prevention (CDC)
<http://www.cdc.gov/>

The CDC is a U.S. federal agency dedicated to disease prevention and control, environmental health, health promotion, and health education. The site features Health Topics A-Z, Data and Statistics, Publications, and a Traveler's Health section. The Traveler's Health section features up-to-date information about destinations, outbreaks, diseases, vaccinations, safe food and water, traveling with children, traveling with pets, special-needs travelers, cruise ships and air travel, and other useful information.

Centre for Arctic Medicine
<http://thule.oulu.fi/public_html/Maineng.html>

The University of Oulu's Thule Institute for Northern Research in Finland focuses on the health of persons living in northern regions of the world. The Centre for Arctic Medicine, part of the medical school and recently merged with the Thule Institute, publishes the *International Journal of Circumpolar Health*. Features include the journal and information about the center.

☑ Foreign and Commonwealth Office (FCO)
<http://www.fco.gov.uk/>

The FCO is the United Kingdom's government office responsible for foreign affairs policy. The site features information related to traveling to specific countries, including the political climate, local customs, safety and security, required vaccinations, and contacting British consulates.

Health Protection Agency
<http://www.hpa.org.uk/>

The Health Protection Agency was established in 2003 to reduce "the impact of infectious diseases, chemical hazards, poisons and radiation hazards," for English and Welsh citizens. This new agency combines the expertise of several organizations of the Public Health Laboratory Service, including the Communicable Disease Surveillance Centre and Central Public Health Laboratory; the Centre for Applied Microbiology and Research; the National Focus for Chemical Incidents; the National Poisons Information Service; and the National Health Service (NHS) public health staff responsible for infectious disease control and emergency planning. The site's features include news, publications, and links.

☑ International Association for Medical Assistance to Travellers (IAMAT)
<http://www.iamat.org/>

Founded in 1960, IAMAT is a nonprofit organization devoted to educating the public about health risks, geographic distribution of diseases, immunization requirements, and environmental conditions (see Figure 7.1). IAMAT maintains a network of European- and North American–trained physicians willing to treat travelers who pay fees to belong to IAMAT. The site's features include charts (malaria risk, world immunization, and malaria protection) and useful links.

International Committee of the Red Cross (ICRC)
<http://www.icrc.org/>

The ICRC site features content in the English, French, and Spanish languages. The ICRC's mandate relates to coordinating international relief activities. Site content of interest to travelers includes information about specific war-torn countries.

International Society for Infectious Diseases (ISID)
<http://www.isid.org/about/>

The International Congress on Infectious Diseases (ICID) and the International Federation on Infectious and Parasitic Diseases (IFIPD) merged in 1986 to form the International Society of Infectious Diseases (ISID). ISID's goals include using research to increase the knowledge base of infectious diseases, promoting the professional development of infectious disease personnel, and fostering partnerships that help control and manage infectious diseases worldwide. The site's features include information about programs, publications, and resources.

International Society of Travel Medicine (ISTM)
<http://www.istm.org/>

ISTM is an international organization with more than 1,200 members in fifty-three countries. ISTM "advocates and facilitates

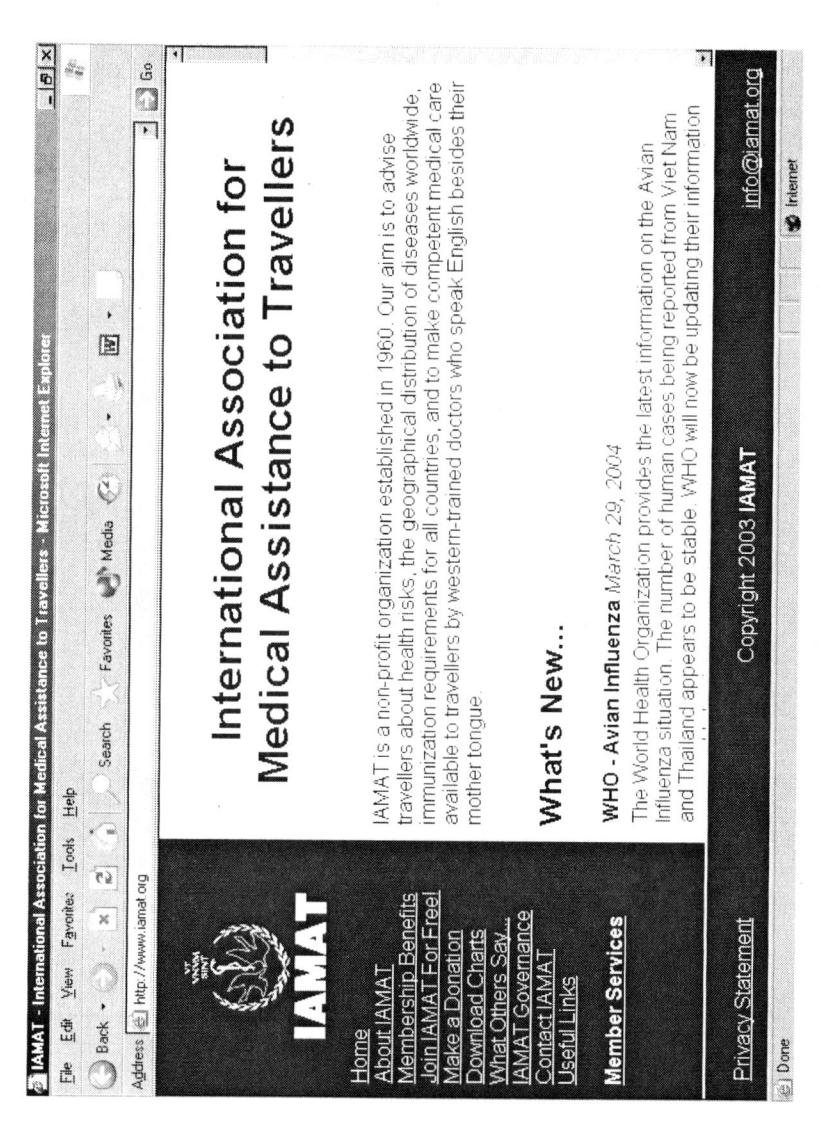

FIGURE 7.1. International Association for Medical Assistance to Travellers (IAMAT) Web Site

education, service, and research activities in the field of travel medicine," including "preventive and curative medicine within many specialties such as tropical medicine, infectious diseases, high altitude physiology, travel related obstetrics, psychiatry, occupational health, military and migration medicine, and environmental health." Site features include educational resources, publications, a Listserv, and news.

National Highway Traffic Safety Administration (NHTSA)
<http://www.nhtsa.dot.gov/>

NHTSA, part of the U.S. Department of Transportation (DOT), provides on its site useful information about airbags, automobile safety, crash statistics, child passenger safety, driver distraction, and other topics.

National Institute of Allergy and Infectious Diseases (NIAID)
<http://www.niaid.nih.gov/default.htm>

NIAID, part of the U.S. National Institutes of Health (NIH), is committed to conducting basic research related to immunology, microbiology, and infectious diseases. Site features include news, activities, and research opportunities.

National Transportation Safety Board (NTSB)
<http://www.ntsb.gov/>

NTSB investigates all civil aviation accidents in the United States, as well as "significant accidents in the other modes of transportation," and issues "safety recommendations aimed at preventing future accidents." NTSB's site features safety information relevant to the aviation, highway, marine, pipeline and hazardous materials, and railroad industries, as well as content on transportation disaster assistance and safety improvements.

Overseas Security Advisory Council (OSAC)
<http://www.ds-osac.org>

The U.S. State Department's OSAC helps exchange information between itself and private-sector corporations and universities, re-

☑ Pan American Health Organization (PAHO)
<http://www.paho.org/>

PAHO works to improve the quality of health for persons living in the countries in the Americas, and serves as a regional office for the World Health Organization (WHO). The site includes information about country-specific health data, vaccines, and immunizations.

Society for Accessible Travel and Hospitality (SATH)
<http://www.sath.org/>

The SATH site features press releases, travel tips, and access information of interest to persons in wheelchairs; those with speech, sight, or hearing impairments; and those with arthritis, diabetes, autism, or kidney disease.

StatePublicHealth.org
<http://www.statepublichealth.org/>

The Robert Wood Johnson Foundation, an organization dedicated to health philanthropy in the United States, provides support for this site. StatePublicHealth.org offers a simple interface to search public health sites; directories of current state health officials, state health agencies, and former state health officials; and public hotlines.

Wilderness Medical Society (WMS)
<http://www.wms.org/>

WMS is devoted to the study of wilderness medicine, a branch of medicine related to "medical problems and treatment in remote environments," including "physiology, clinical medicine, preventive medicine, and public health." The site's features include information about conferences, interest groups, publications, and resources.

☑ World Health Organization (WHO)
<http://www.who.int/>

WHO was established in 1948 as the health agency of the United Nations. Governed by 192 member states through the World Health Assembly, WHO's objective "is the attainment by all peoples of the highest possible level of health." Site features include publications, health topics, and research tools.

Chapter 8

Full-Text Publications

Many educational, governmental, and commercial sites include full-text documents related to travel health. Publications posted in portable document format (PDF) require installation of Adobe Acrobat software (available free from <http://www.adobe.com/>) to view, download, or print the documents. The symbol ☑ is used to denote major resources that can be used to seek authoritative and original content on aspects of travel health.

☑ *Air Travel Consumer Report*
<http://airconsumer.ost.dot.gov/report.htm>

Published by the U.S. Department of Transportation (DOT), this monthly report includes information about flight delays, mishandled baggage, oversales, and consumer complaints.

Art of Travel
<http://www.artoftravel.com/>

Written by John Gregory, *Art of Travel* covers several topics of interest to travelers, including water purification, effects of the sun, traveling alone, and food poisoning.

☑ *"Bad Bug Book"*
<http://vm.cfsan.fda.gov/~mow/intro.html>

This publication, issued by the Center for Food Safety and Applied Nutrition, a department of the U.S. Food and Drug Administration (FDA), includes useful information about food-borne pathogenic microorganisms (bacteria, viruses, and parasites) and natural toxins that cause diseases in humans (see Figure 8.1). Typical entries feature the name of the organism or group of organisms, nature of acute disease, nature of disease (acute symptoms, onset time, infective dose, duration of symptoms, and cause of disease), diagnosis of human illness, associated foods, relative frequency of disease, reported cases, complications, susceptible populations, foods analysis, selected outbreaks, education, and other resources. The *"Bad Bug Book"* is also called *Foodborne Pathogenic Microorganisms and Natural Toxins Handbook*.

Biosecurity and Bioterrorism: Biodefense Strategy, Practice, and Science
<http://www.medscape.com/viewpublication/907_index>

First released in 2003 by publisher Mary Ann Liebert and accessible through Medscape, this quarterly publication is "dedicated to bioscience, medical and public health response, infrastructure and institutions, international collaborations, agroterror/food safety, and citizen response and responsibility, as each of these issues relate to biodefense." Typical articles address issues such as aerosol dissemination of biological weapons, anthrax, and other topics. Medscape requires free registration.

☑ *Bulletin of the World Health Organization: The International Journal of Public Health*
<http://www.who.int/bulletin/>

Bulletin of the World Health Organization is published monthly, featuring "public health information of international significance." Past journal issues have included articles about malnutrition, diarrhea, malaria, and other topics.

☑ *Canada Communicable Disease Report (CCDR)*
<http://www.hc-sc.gc.ca/pphb-dgspsp/publicat/ccdr-rmtc/index.html>

Health Canada's Population and Public Health Branch (PPHB) publishes this report and provides free access to *Canada Communicable Disease Report (CCDR)* issues dating from 1995 to the

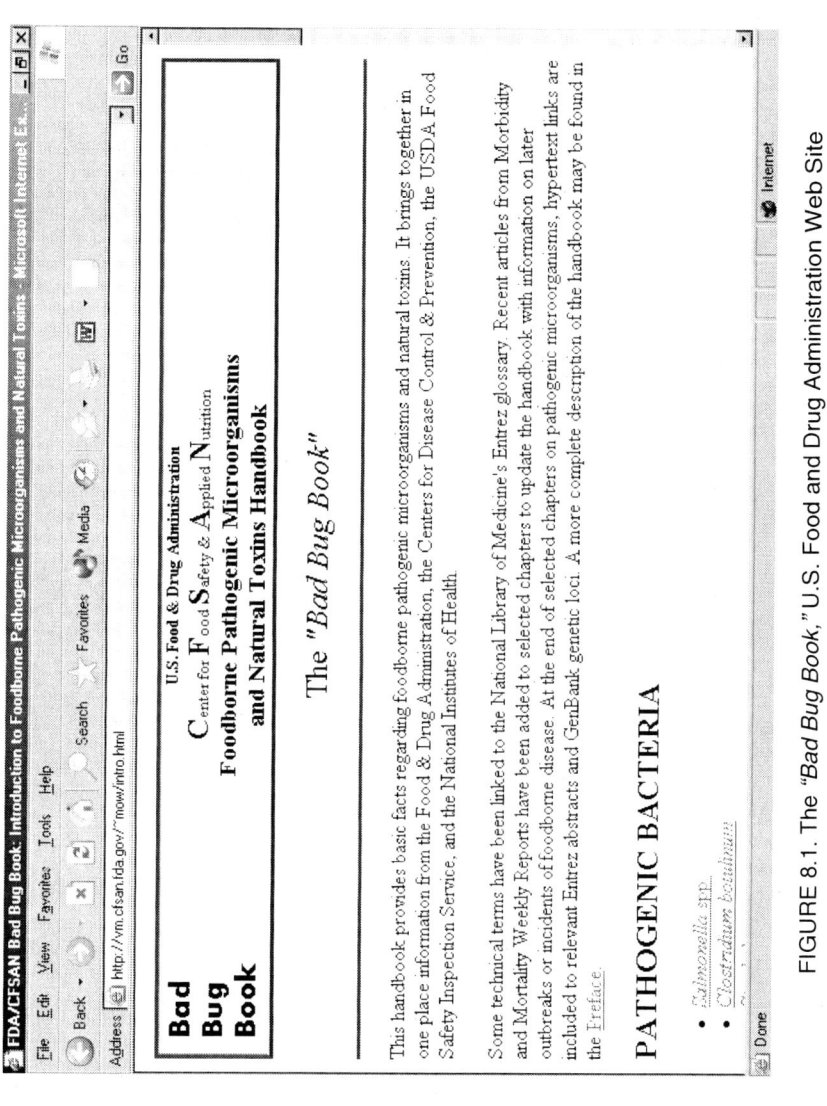

FIGURE 8.1. The *"Bad Bug Book,"* U.S. Food and Drug Administration Web Site

present. Typical issues include information about severe acute respiratory syndrome (SARS), tuberculosis, hepatitis C, and other topics of potential interest to travelers. Advisory committee statements and supplements to the *CCDR* include up-to-date information about topics such as jet lag, immunization recommendations for persons with cochlear implants, and information about vaccines with mercury-based preservatives.

☑ **CDC "Blue Sheet"**
<http://www.cdc.gov/travel/blusheet.htm>

Commonly known as the "Blue Sheet," the *Summary of Health Information for International Travel,* as developed by the U.S. Centers for Disease Control and Prevention (CDC), lists cholera-infected countries, yellow fever–infected countries, plague-infected countries, outbreak notices, travel alerts, and travel advisories.

☑ **CDC *Fact Book 2000/2001***
<http://www.cdc.gov/maso/factbook/main.htm>

Although not geared specifically toward travel health, the Centers for Disease Control and Prevention's (CDC) *Fact Book 2000/2001* includes information about plans to improve health and prevent AIDS in Africa and India; food-borne diseases; hepatitis A, B, and C; influenza; and other diseases (see Figure 8.2).

☑ **CDC "Green Sheet"**
<http://www2.cdc.gov/nceh/vsp/VSP_RptGreenSheet.asp>

The U.S. Centers for Disease Control and Prevention (CDC) publishes the *Summary of Sanitation Inspections of International Cruise Ships,* also known as the "Green Sheet." This publication lists ships by name, inspection date, and score. Sanitation standards cover water; food preparation and holding; potential contamination of food; and general cleanliness, storage, and repair.

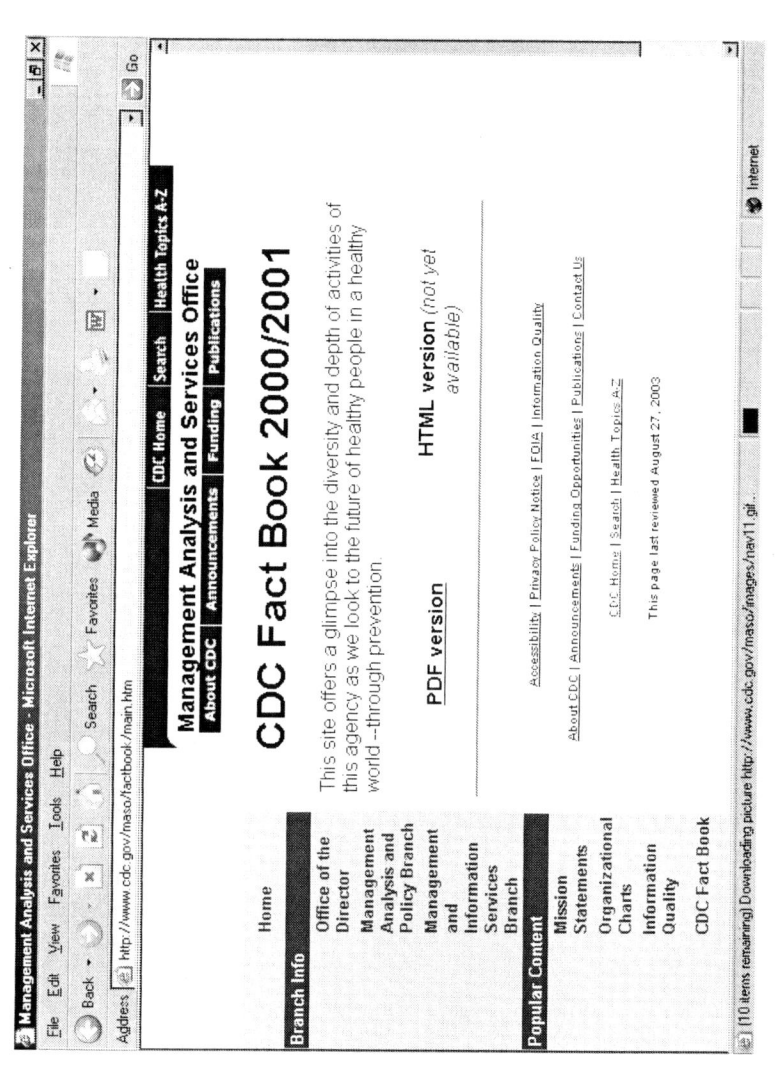

FIGURE 8.2. CDC *Fact Book 2000/2001*, U.S. Centers for Disease Control and Prevention (CDC) Web Site

119

CDR Weekly
<http://www.hpa.org.uk/cdr/default.htm>

CDR Weekly, previously published by the United Kingdom's Public Health Laboratory Services, is now published by the recently organized Health Protection Agency. *CDR Weekly* is an electronic bulletin published every Thursday, that features public health news; epidemiological data; and reports related to bacteremia, respiratory and enteric illnesses, HIV, sexually transmitted diseases, immunizations, and zoonotic diseases.

Clinical Infectious Diseases—News
<http://www.journals.uchicago.edu/CID/journal/news.html>

Although *Clinical Infectious Diseases*, published by the University of Chicago, is available to paid subscribers only, the journal's site features a freely accessible news section that includes information about topics such as HIV prevention, HIV testing, smallpox vaccines, severe acute respiratory syndrome (SARS) precautions, Ebola virus, and other subjects.

☑ Disease Outbreak News
<http://www.who.int/csr/don/en/>

The Communicable Disease Surveillance and Response (CSR) department of the World Health Organization (WHO) publishes *Disease Outbreak News* as a medium for disseminating information to contain known risks, respond to unexpected health threats, and improve preparedness throughout the world. Archived issues from 1996 to the present can be sorted by disease, year, and country.

Disease Surveillance On-Line
<http://www.hc-sc.gc.ca/pphb-dgspsp/dsol-smed/index.html>

Health Canada's Population and Public Health Branch (PPHB) created this Web-based resource to help disseminate surveillance data related to notifiable diseases from AIDS to yellow fever. Typical entries include information such as agent of disease, worldwide distribution, symptoms, period of communicability, mode of transmission, prevention, and related links.

Drugs and Travel: Why They Don't Mix
<http://www.voyage.gc.ca/main/pubs/PDF/drugs_travel-en.pdf>

This ten-page booklet was developed by Canada's Department of Foreign Affairs and Foreign Trade. Advice includes what to do if arrested, how to carry legal medications when traveling, the effects of illicit drugs, and assistance from the Canadian government.

Elderly Travel
<http://www.traveldoc.com/info/elderlytravel.asp>

The International Medicine Center (IMC), which hosts the TravelDoc site, prepared this two-page document about the risks of travel by the elderly.

☑ Emerging Infectious Diseases
<http://www.cdc.gov/ncidod/EID/>

The National Center for Infectious Diseases, part of the U.S. Centers for Disease Control and Prevention (CDC), publishes *Emerging Infectious Diseases* as a means to distribute information about evolving and changing disease patterns. Site features include expedited content, e-mail notifications of updated content, announcements about conferences, and content translated into Chinese, French, and Spanish. The content is peer reviewed.

☑ Emporiatrics: An Introduction to Travel Medicine
<http://www.vh.org/adult/provider/internalmedicine/TravelMedicine/TravelMedHP.html>

First published in 1993 and revised in 2000, this work provides practical information about immunizations, prevention of travel-related diseases, travelers with special conditions (pregnancy, disabilities, diabetes, heart diseases, chronic lung diseases, HIV), traveling with children, general precautions and advice, recommendations for travel to specific regions, and sources of information and reference. The work's physician editors are associated with Virginia Commonwealth University.

Epidemiological Bulletin
   <http://www.paho.org/English/SHA/beindexe.htm>

The Pan American Health Organization (PAHO), an international organization based in Washington, DC, is dedicated to improving "health and living standards of the people of the Americas," and strengthening "national and local health systems . . . in collaboration with Ministries of Health, other government and international agencies, nongovernmental organizations, universities, social security agencies, community groups, and many others." PAHO provides access to issues of the quarterly *Epidemiological Bulletin* from 1990 to the present.

EPI-News
   <http://www2.state.tn.us/health/CEDS/epi.htm>

Communicable and Environmental Disease Services, a division of the Tennessee Department of Health publishes this quarterly newsletter. Information includes disease occurrence and notifiable diseases within the state.

Eurosurveillance Monthly and *Eurosurveillance Weekly*
   <http://www.eurosurveillance.org/index-02.asp>

The European Commission funds the Eurosurveillance Project "to promote the diffusion and exchange of information on communicable diseases." Publications include *Eurosurveillance,* which is published monthly, and a weekly bulletin, *Eurosurveillance Weekly. Eurosurveillance Monthly* is peer reviewed and includes "original articles on the epidemiology of communicable diseases, surveillance reports, comparisons between the national public health policies in Europe, and outbreaks investigation reports."

Eurosurveillance Weekly includes epidemic alerts, updates, and responses, as well as new information about infectious diseases and surveillance data. Free registration entitles subscribers to free updates sent by e-mail.

Foodborne Pathogenic Microorganisms and Natural Toxins Handbook
<http://vm.cfsan.fda.gov/percent7Emow/intro.html>

Published in 1992 by the Center for Food Safety and Applied Nutrition, a department of the U.S. Food and Drug Administration (FDA), this handbook (also called The *"Bad Bug Book"*) includes useful information about food-borne pathogenic microorganisms (bacteria, viruses, and parasites) and natural toxins that can cause diseases in humans. Typical entries feature the name of the organism or group of organisms, nature of disease (acute symptoms, onset time, infective dose, duration of symptoms, and cause of disease), diagnosis of human illness, associated foods, relative frequency of disease, reported cases, complications, susceptible populations, foods analysis, selected outbreaks, education, and other resources.

☑ Guidelines for Vaccinating Pregnant Women
<http://www.cdc.gov/nip/publications/preg_guide.htm>

Although the National Immunization Program section of the U.S. Centers for Disease Control and Prevention (CDC) emphasizes routine child and adult immunization schedules, the site also includes information useful to pregnant women planning to travel to areas that require additional immunizations. This fifteen-page guide was updated in October 2003.

☑ Health Advice for Travellers
<http://www.dh.gov.uk/PolicyandGuidance/HealthAdviceToTravellers/fs/en>

The British Department of Health (DOH) developed this handy guide that covers world health risks, travel planning, and treatment while traveling. The risk information explains the need for immunizations, food and drink precautions, outdoor safety, and more. The planning information discusses the need for checkups, first aid kits, insurance, etc. The treatment information covers Form E111, a document that allows citizens of European Economic Area (EEA) countries to seek emergency medical treatment in most European countries.

Hints for Staying Healthy: HIV and Travel
<http://www.anacnet.org/media/docs/hiv-nurse/hiv-nurse_spring2001.pdf>

The Association of Nurses in AIDS Care (ANAC) publishes this newsletter for HIV-positive individuals. The Spring 2001 issue focuses on staying healthy while traveling and includes a chart of recommended vaccines.

Infections in Medicine
<http://www.medscape.com/viewpublication/91_index>

Issues from 1998 to the present are accessible through Medscape, which requires free registration. *Infections in Medicine* "provides the clinician with practical reports on prevention, diagnosis, public health issues, and treatment. Issues concerning cost-effectiveness and infection control are regularly addressed."

Infectious Diseases News Brief
<http://www.hc-sc.gc.ca/pphb-dgspsp/bid-bmi/dsd-dsm/nb-ab/index.html>

The Population and Public Health Branch (PPHB) of Health Canada provides "a weekly digest of national and international information about communicable disease incidents and issues." Examples of diseases covered include influenza in Canada, shigellosis in Texas, and cholera in Iraq.

International Journal of Circumpolar Health
<http://ijch.oulu.fi/>

Finland's International Union for Circumpolar Health, Nordic Society of Circumpolar Health, and the University of Oulu publish this journal to distribute information about health issues faced by peoples living in circumpolar regions. Although the journal is not geared toward travel health, persons planning to travel to the Arctic region may be interested in some of the topics.

☑ *International Travel and Health*
<http://www.who.int/ith/>

Redesigned in 2002, this World Health Organization (WHO) resource provides useful information about the cause, transmission, geographical distribution, risk for travelers, prevention, and precautions for specific diseases from anthrax to yellow fever. Other topics include travel by air; environmental health risks; infectious diseases; vaccine-preventable diseases; malaria; blood transfusions; accidents, injuries, and violence; and other topics. Additional features include a checklist for travelers and disease maps for cholera, dengue fever, hepatitis, HIV, malaria, encephalitis, polio, rabies, tuberculosis, and yellow fever.

The Internet Journal of Infectious Diseases
<http://www.ispub.com/ostia/index.php?xmlFilePath= journals/ijid/current.xml>

This peer-reviewed publication includes scholarly articles on the subject of infectious diseases. The editor-in-chief is Stephen B. Kennedy, a physician with a master's degree in public health.

☑ *Medical Guidelines for Airline Travel*
<http://www.asma.org/Publication/medguid.pdf>

The Aerospace Medical Association (ASMA) publishes this twenty-two-page publication that is in its second edition (see Figure 8.3). The document covers stressors of flight; medical evaluation; in-flight medical care; first aid kits; recommended immunizations and malaria prevention; cardiovascular contraindications to commercial air travel; pregnancy and air travel; ear, nose, and throat diseases; surgical conditions; psychiatric conditions; and other ailments.

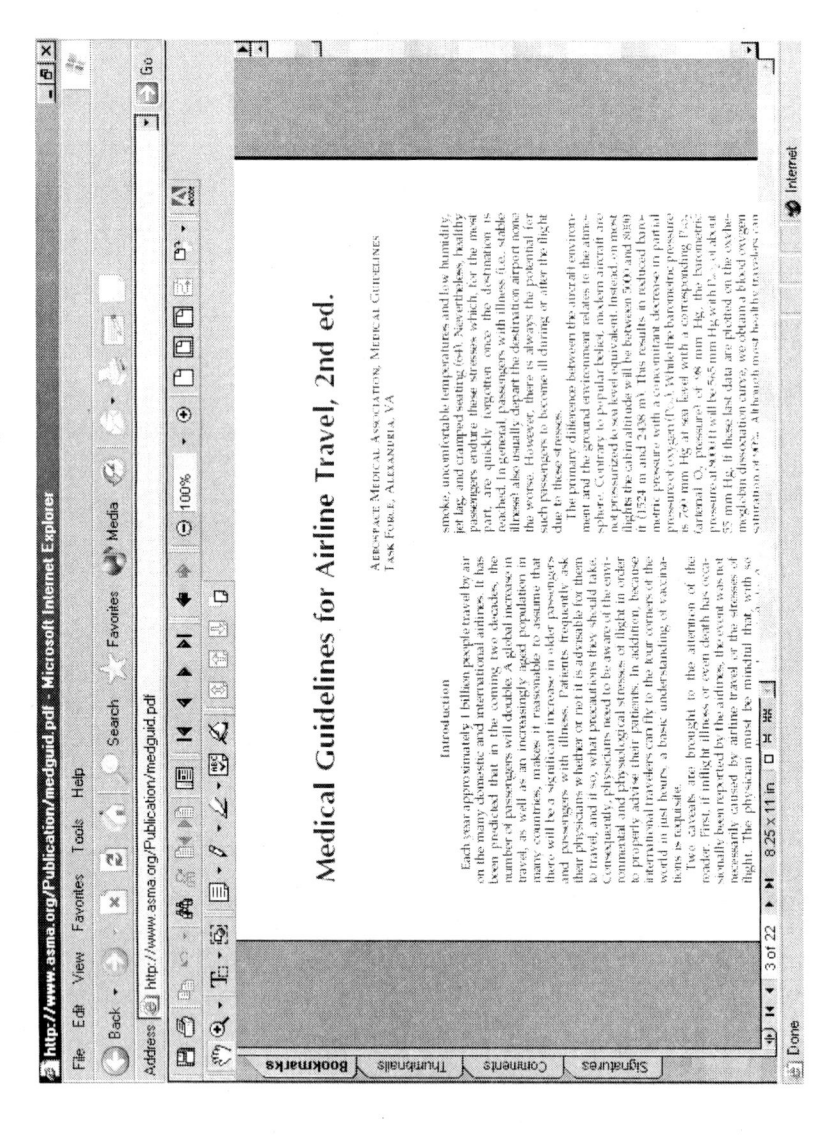

FIGURE 8.3. *Medical Guidelines for Airline Travel*, Aerospace Medical Association Web Site

☑ *Morbidity and Mortality Weekly Report (MMWR)*
  <http://www.cdc.gov/mmwr/mmwr_wk.html>

The U.S. Centers for Disease Control and Prevention (CDC) provides free access to its weekly report of data submitted to the CDC by state and territorial health departments in the United States (see Figure 8.4). The information published in *MMWR* is considered provisional and covers "reports on infectious and chronic diseases, environmental hazards, natural or human-generated disasters, occupational diseases and injuries, and intentional and unintentional injuries," as well as "topics of international interest and notices of events of interest to the public health community."

Out on a Limb: Advice for the Adventure Traveller
  <http://www.voyage.gc.ca/main/pubs/PDF/out_on_limb-en.asp>

Canada's Department of Foreign Affairs and International Trade developed this five-page document for adventure travelers.

SARS Reference
  <http://sarsreference.com/>

Developed by Bernd Sebastian Kamps and Christian Hoffmann in May 2003, this resource promises to be updated monthly during the duration of the severe acute respiratory syndrome (SARS) epidemic. This e-book includes a timeline of the disease, as well as information about the disease's virology, transmission, prevention, epidemiology, case definition, diagnostic tests, clinical presentation, diagnosis, treatment, and SARS in children.

Travelling Abroad? Assistance for Canadians
  <http://www.voyage.gc.ca/main/pubs/PDF/travelling_abroad-en.pdf>

Canada's Department of Foreign Affairs and International Trade developed this one-page document for Canadian travelers. The brochure explains the role of consular services to assist citizens traveling abroad.

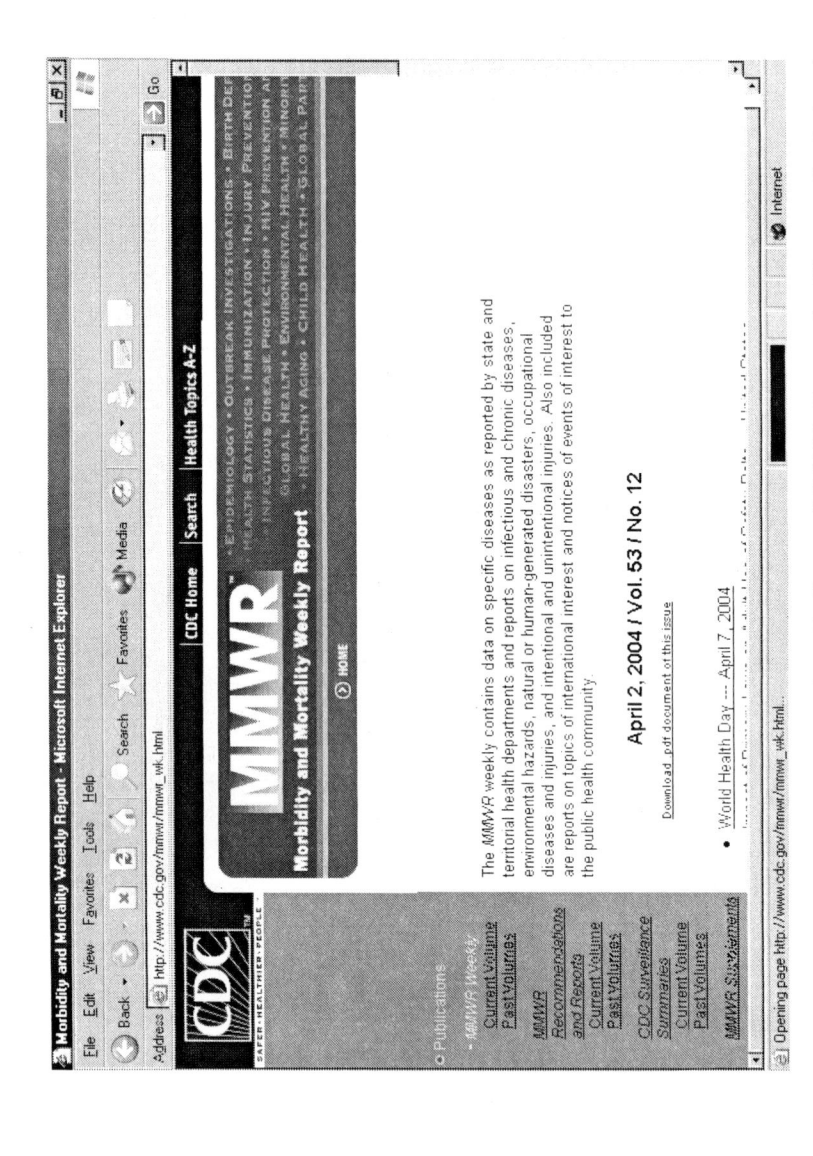

FIGURE 8.4. *Morbidity and Mortality Weekly Report (MMWR)*, Centers for Disease Control and Prevention (CDC) Web Site

Tropical Medicine and Hygiene News
<http://www.astmh.org/newsltr.asp>

Published by the American Society of Tropical Medicine and Hygiene (ASTMH), this bimonthly newsletter features information about disease trends, legislative news, conferences, funding opportunities, and more.

☑ Tuberculosis and Air Travel
<http://www.who.int/gtb/publications/aircraft/>

The World Health Organization (WHO) publishes *Tuberculosis and Air Travel: Guidelines for Prevention and Control.*

Victorian Infectious Diseases Bulletin
<http://www.dhs.vic.gov.au/phb/vidb/current.htm>

The State Government of Victoria in Australia publishes this quarterly bulletin to provide "summaries of infectious diseases surveillance data, local news, outbreak investigations, infection control procedures, clinical cases of general interest and brief reports on original clinical or laboratory based research."

☑ Weekly Epidemiological Record
<http://www.who.int/wer/>

The electronic version of the World Health Organization's (WHO) *Weekly Epidemiological Record (WER)* is available free of charge. *WER* "serves as an essential instrument for the rapid and accurate dissemination of epidemiological information on cases and outbreaks of diseases under the International Health Regulations and on other communicable diseases of public health importance, including the newly emerging or reemerging infections."

☑ World Factbook
<http://www.odci.gov/cia/publications/factbook/>

Published annually by the U.S. Central Intelligence Agency (CIA), with some content, such as maps, updated more frequently, this handy resource includes country-specific data about geography, people, government, economy, communications, transportation, military, and transnational issues (see Figure 8.5). This work also includes maps and flags of the world.

World Health Report: Reducing Risks, Promoting Healthy Life
<http://www.who.int/whr/en/>

Published yearly in all six World Health Organization (WHO) languages (English, French, Spanish, Arabic, Chinese, and Russian), this report "measures the amount of disease, disability and death in the world today" and determines how many diseases can be reduced or avoided over the next twenty years.

☑ World Immunization Chart
<http://www.iamat.org/pdf/WorldImmunization.pdf>

Published by the International Association for Medical Assistance to Travellers (IAMAT) and frequently updated, this publication lists required and recommended immunizations for travel to specific countries; immunizations specific to travelers such as Muslim pilgrims and contract workers; and the geographic distribution of hepatitis B, Japanese encephalitis, rabies, plague, tick-borne encephalitis, and yellow fever.

World Malaria Risk Chart
<http://www.iamat.org/pdf/WorldMalariaRisk.pdf>

Published by the International Association for Medical Assistance to Travellers (IAMAT) and frequently updated, this publication lists the relative risk of malaria in specific countries alphabetically from Afghanistan to Zimbabwe, as well as malaria-free countries.

☑ The "Yellow Book": Health Information for International Travel, 2003-2004
<http://www.cdc.gov/travel/yb/index.htm>

Although the U.S. Centers for Disease Control and Prevention (CDC) sells copies of this publication, the book's content is also

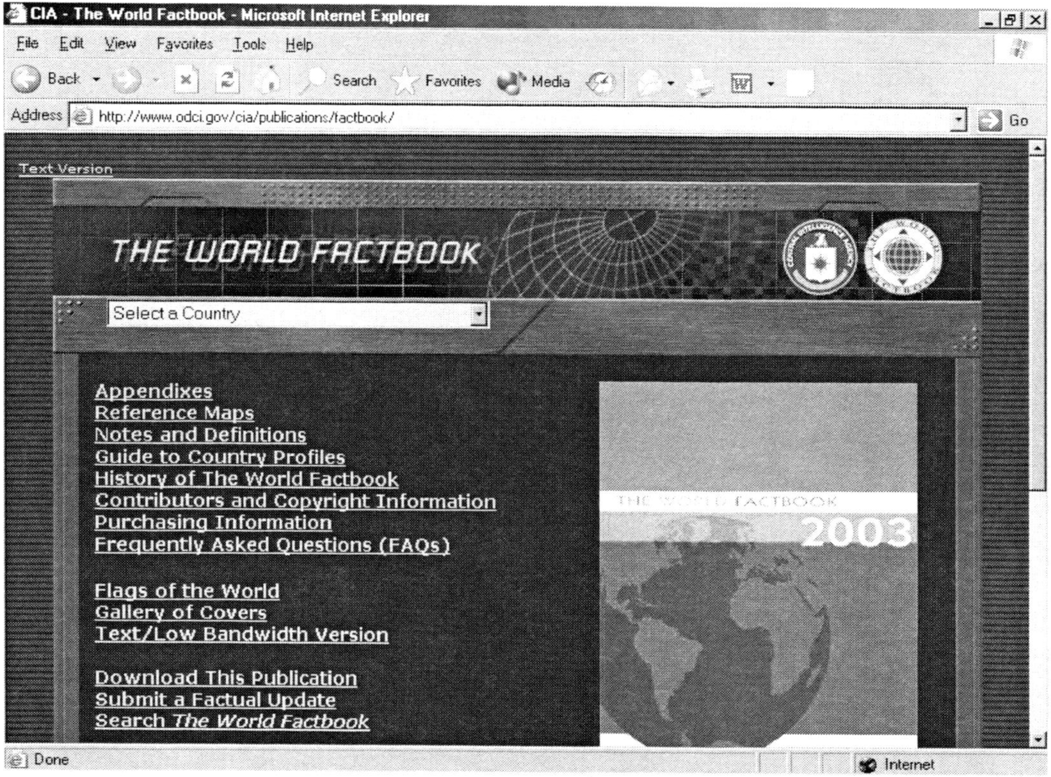

FIGURE 8.5. *World Factbook 2003*, U.S. Central Intelligence Agency (CIA) Web Site

featured on its site (see Figure 8.6). Chapters cover vaccinations, health hints for international travelers, geographic distribution of specific health hazards, travelers with special needs, traveling with children, and more.

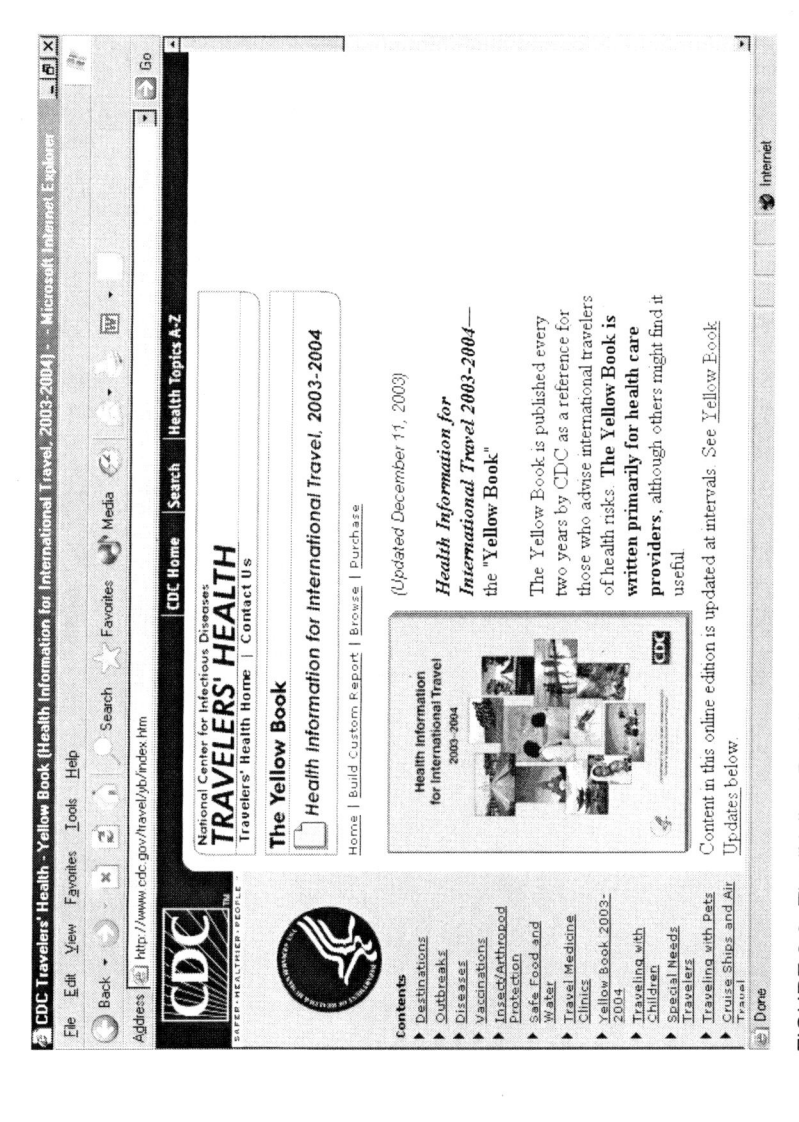

FIGURE 8.6. *The "Yellow Book": Health Information for International Travel, 2003-2004*, Centers for Disease Control and Prevention (CDC) Web Site

133

Glossary

Some of the terms used throughout this guide may be unfamiliar to the layperson. These definitions were derived from several excellent sources:

- **Dictionary.com**
  <http://dictionary.reference.com/>
- **Hyperdictionary**
  <http://www.hyperdictionary.com/>
- **medical-dictionary.com**
  <http://www.medical-dictionary.com/>
- **MedlinePlus Medical Dictionary**
  <http://www.nlm.nih.gov/medlineplus/mplusdictionary.html>
- **MedTerms.com Medical Dictionary**
  <http://www.medterms.com/>
- **OneLook Dictionary Search**
  <http://beta.onelook.com/>

aggregated: Collected or combined.

allergy: A high sensitivity to irritants, such as pollens, foods, or microorganisms, resulting in physical reactions in the afflicted person.

amebiasis: An infection or disease caused by amebas (protozoan organisms) that can cause diarrheal illness. Amebiasis is often caused by the *Entamoeba histolytica* organism.

anaphylaxis: An immediate and severe allergic reaction that sometimes results in shock and death.

anatomical: Related to the structure of an organism, such as a human or animal.

antibody: Protein that develops after the introduction of an antigen that can protect the body from a specific disease.

antigen: A substance used to stimulate an immune response.

antitoxin: An antibody capable of neutralizing or reducing the action of a toxin.

arthropods: A group of insects that includes crustaceans (lobster, crab, shrimp, barnacle), arachnids (spider, scorpion, mite, tick), and myriapods (centipede, millipede) with hard exterior skeletons, segmented bodies, and jointed legs.

bacteria: Microscopic organisms that can cause disease.

bibliography: A list of citations that include author, title, source, and abstract, all of which is useful information for finding full-text information in print or electronic publications.

biologicals: Therapeutic substances made from living organisms; examples include vaccines, antitoxins, sera, and globulins.

blood-borne: Carried or transmitted by contact with blood or blood transfusion.

"Blue Sheet": The common name for the *Summary of Health Information for International Travel,* a work developed by the U.S. Centers for Disease Control and Prevention (CDC).

bovine: Pertaining to an ox, cow, or buffalo.

channel: As related to a Web site, a specific subsection of content. One site may have several channels devoted to specific topics or audiences.

chemoprophylaxis: The use of drugs to prevent disease. *See also* PROPHYLAXIS.

circadian rhythms: Biological processes that occur at twenty-four-hour intervals.

circumpolar: Located in one of the polar regions (Arctic, Antarctic).

Glossary

clinical trial: Series of treatments used to evaluate the effectiveness of specific medications or medical procedures.

communicable diseases: Diseases that are contagious or easily transmitted from one organism to another.

consular information sheet: Publication with location of embassy offices in a specific country, health conditions, political instabilities, criminal activities, and other information useful to travelers.

consulate: Office or building that serves as the workplace for embassy staff.

contraindication: A condition or disease that makes a particular treatment or procedure inadvisable.

degenerative: Causing deterioration or loss of function.

desynchronosis: Jet lag.

diagnosis: The process of identifying characteristics, signs, or symptoms of a disease, condition, or ailment to distinguish the disease from other diseases.

disease surveillance: Close observation and tracking of disease activity by public health authorities. *See also* SURVEILLANCE.

disease vectors: Organisms such as mosquitoes or ticks that carry disease-causing microorganisms from one host (person or animal) to another.

diuretics: Substances that increase the flow of urine.

e-book: The electronic format or version of a printed book, or a distinct publication available only on disk or online.

ecotourism: Travel that emphasizes ecology and natural flora and fauna.

embassy: The office of a foreign government, headed by an ambassador.

emetophobia: Fear of vomiting.

emporiatrics: A medical specialty that focuses on medical aspects of travel.

encephalopathy: A degenerative disease of the brain.

endemic: Prevalent in or peculiar to a specific geographic region.

enteric: Related to or within the intestine.

epidemic: The outbreak and spread of disease in a geographic area.

etiology: The study of the causes of disease.

fauna: Animals living in a specific region.

flora: Plants growing in a specific region.

food-borne: Carried or caused by foods or beverages.

gastroenteritis: Stomach or intestinal upset, including nausea, vomiting, and diarrhea, often caused by food poisoning.

globulin: A protein found in blood, milk, muscle, and plant seeds.

gray literature: Publications that are not widely available through normal channels.

"Green Sheet": Informal name for the U.S. Centers for Disease Control and Prevention's (CDC) *Summary of Sanitation Inspections of International Cruise Ships.*

health tourism: Travel to an overseas location for the purpose of obtaining medical procedures, surgery, treatment, or recuperation.

hemorrhagic: Characterized by sudden and/or excessive loss of blood.

hepatitis: Inflammation of the liver caused by infection or toxins.

homeopathy: Medical practice based on the principle of "like cures like"; the use of tiny amounts of drugs that mimic the symptoms of the disease being treated.

hyperthermia: Abnormally high body temperature.

hypothermia: Abnormally low body temperature.

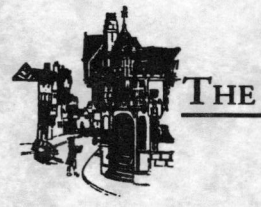

THE HAWORTH PRESS, INC.

For your review with our compliments

For additional information, comments, or to send tearsheets:

Shelley Jones, Book Review Coordinator
email: sjones@HaworthPress.com

10 Alice Street, Binghamton, NY 13904–1580 USA
Tel: (607) 722–5857 • Fax: (607) 722–6362
Email: getinfo@HaworthPress.com • Web: www.HaworthPress.com

immune response: Response to an antigen by a specific antibody.

immunization: A procedure that introduces specific antigens to induce an immune response, thereby improving the ability to resist infection; introduction of harmless or killed bacterial or viral organisms to render immunity for a specific disease. *Compare* VACCINATION.

immunocompromised: The lack of a normal immune response, resulting from disease, malnutrition, or immunosuppressive therapy.

MEDLINE: A bibliographic database of the published biomedical literature developed by the U.S. National Library of Medicine (NLM).

microorganisms: Tiny life forms such as bacteria or protozoa.

morbidity: Relative incidence or rate of disease.

mortality: Relative incidence or rate of death.

mycobacteria: A type of bacteria, some of which cause tuberculosis and leprosy.

mycotic: Related to infections or diseases caused by fungus.

notifiable diseases: Diseases required by law to be reported to public health authorities.

occurrence: Instances of diseases appearing in a population.

ostomy: A surgically created opening, such as a tracheostomy, ileostomy, or colostomy.

otolaryngology: A branch of medicine that focuses on diseases of the ear, nose, and throat.

outbreak: Sudden increase or eruption of disease.

parasite: An organism that feeds on another organism often called the host.

pathogen: An agent or substance than can cause disease.

peer review: Professional evaluation of a colleague's work.

philanthropy: Activities and monetary donations intended to improve the well-being of others.

phlebitis: Inflammation of a vein. *See also* THROMBOPHLEBITIS.

portal: As related to Web sites, a gateway of resources.

prophylaxis: Protective or preventive measures taken to prevent specific diseases.

protozoa: Single-celled organisms, including amoebas, ciliates, flagellates, and sporozoans.

public announcement: A type of written communication used by the U.S. State Department to inform American citizens about terrorism threats and other short-term conditions that affect safety and security while traveling to or living in other countries.

quarantine: Enforced isolation of potentially contagious individuals or animals to prevent the spread of disease.

search directory: A Web tool that organizes Internet resources by subject and/or file type (documents, images, news group messages).

search engine: A Web tool that finds Internet resources based on keywords or phrases typed into a search interface.

seroconversion: The body's development of antibodies in reaction to antigens.

serum: A constituent part of blood; often contains antibodies.

special needs: In this context, refers to persons with physical differences or disabilities that affect comfort or mobility while traveling.

spongiform: Having a soft, porous, and spongelike texture.

stent: A thin thread or rod used to support the inside of a blood vessel or other anatomical structure.

surveillance: Close observations of persons or situations. *See also* DISEASE SURVEILLANCE.

Glossary

thrombophlebitis: Inflammation of a blood vessel with a blood clot. *See also* PHLEBITIS.

thrombosis: The formation of a blood clot in a blood vessel.

tick-borne: Carried or transmitted by ticks.

tissue: As related to the body, a collection of similar cells that act together and perform specific functions.

toxin: Harmful substance that can cause disease.

transmission: Transfer of a disease from one person or animal to another.

travel warning: A written communication issued by the U.S. State Department recommending that American citizens avoid or curtail travel to a specific country or region.

tropical: Related to regions located in the tropics, hot and humid areas that are twenty-three degrees, twenty-seven feet north or south of the Earth's equator.

ultraviolet (UV) rays: Invisible light from the sun that can cause sunburn and skin damage.

vaccination: Introduction of harmless or killed bacterial or viral organisms to render immunity for a specific disease; a procedure that introduces specific antigens to induce an immune response, thereby improving the ability to resist infection. *Compare* IMMUNIZATION.

vaccines: Preparations of microorganisms used to stimulate an immune response to prevent future infection with similar microorganisms.

vector: A tick, mosquito, or other organism that transports disease-carrying microorganisms from one host to another.

viruses: Submicroscopic organisms that infect plants, animals, and humans, often causing diseases.

Web browser: A software program, such as Netscape or Internet Explorer, used to view content (text, images) on the World Wide Web.

white paper: An authoritative report on an issue of concern or controversy.

"Yellow Book": Also known as *Health Information for International Travel*, published by the U.S. Centers for Disease Control and Prevention (CDC).

zoonosis: Disease transmitted from animals to humans (also known as "zoonotic disease").

Suggested Readings

Chiodini, Jane and Boyne, Lorna. *Atlas of Travel Medicine and Health*. Hamilton, Ontario, Canada: B.C. Decker, 2003.

Coleman, Marlene. *Safe and Sound: Health Travel with Children*. Guilford, CT: Globe Pequot Press, 2003.

Jong, Elaine C. *The Travel and Tropical Medicine Manual*. Philadelphia, PA: Saunders, 2003.

Keystone, Jay S., Kozarsky, Phyllis, Freedman, David O., Nothdurft, Hans D., and Connor, Bradley A. *Travel Medicine*. St. Louis, MO: Mosby, 2003.

Shannon, Joyce Brennfleck. *Traveler's Health Sourcebook*. Detroit, MI: Omnigraphics, 2000.

Steffen, Robert. *Manual of Travel Medicine and Health*. Hamilton, Ontario, Canada: B.C. Decker, 2003.

Wilks, Jeff and Page, Stephen. *Managing Tourist Health and Safety in the New Millennium*. Amsterdam, the Netherlands: Pergamon, 2003.

Index

Page numbers followed by the letter "f" indicate figures; those followed by the letter "t" indicate tables.

Accidents
    air crashes, 35-36, 101, 112
    automobile fatalities, 45
    bus crashes, 107-108
    prevention, 35
    statistics, 37, 39, 45, 112
    traffic safety, 35-37, 99, 112
    train fatalities, 39
Adventure travel, 127
Aerospace medicine, 125, 126f
AIDS/HIV
    HIV-positive travelers, 26, 83, 124
    testing requirements, 25, 83
    vaccinations, 26, 28, 124
Air
    quality, 101, 103, 105
    rage, 65-66
Air travel
    children, traveling with, 7, 40, 41
    children traveling alone, 40, 41
    consumer complaints, 115
    crashes, 35-36, 101
    flight delays, 15
    pets, 53-57
    traffic control, 101
Allergies, 66-67, 112
Altitude
    effects on ears, 78
    sickness, 13, 14, 16, 68
Amebiasis, 77-78
Anaphylaxis, 66-67
Anxiety related to flying, 80
Arctic medicine, 71, 109, 124-125

Arthritis, 68-69
Asthma, 66, 67
Automobile driving
    accident prevention, 35
    behavior, 65-66, 102
    directions, 103
    disabled drivers, 45-46
    distance calculators, 103
    evacuation safety, 48
    fatalities, 45
    international, 36, 37
    maps, 37, 103
    with pets, 53-57
    safety, 35, 36, 37, 99, 112
    tests, 37, 102
    traffic congestion reports, 104
    winter weather, 36

Back pain, 12, 69-70
Biologicals, 28
Biosecurity, 116
Bioterrorism, 116
Birds, 53-57, 58f
Bites and stings
    insects, 70-71, 95-96
    marine life, 71
Blizzards, automobile driving, 36
Bovine spongiform encephalopathy, 89
Breast-feeding, 92
British Department of Health, 10, 12, 23, 24f

145

British Foreign and Commonwealth
    Office, 10, 17, 96, 109
Browser software, 1, 4
Bugs. *See* Insects
Bureau of Consular Affairs (United
    States), 18, 19f, 20, 37, 52
Bus travel
    children traveling alone, 40
    children traveling with, 40-41
    international, 107-108
    with pets, 53
    safety, 39, 107-108

Calculators
    driving distance, 103
    jet lag, 13, 102-103
Car driving. *See* Automobile driving
Cardiovascular diseases, 88
Cats, 53-57, 58f
Certificates, health, 23, 25, 26, 27, 53, 56
Checklists, 23, 25-26, 31
Children
    allergies, 67
    asthma, 67
    diabetes mellitus, 31
    Lyme disease, 88-89
    safety seats, 35, 99
    SARS, 127
    sun-related ailments, 94-95
    traveling alone, 40, 41
    traveling with, 7, 40, 41
Cholera, 118, 124, 125
Circumpolar medicine, 71-72, 109,
    124-125
Climate, 99, 100f, 101
Clot disorders, 7, 72-73, 74f, 75
Cold weather illnesses, 71-72
Consular services
    Canada, 127, 108
    United Kingdom, 10, 109
    United States, 18, 19f, 20, 45, 52
Consumer health, 7, 8, 101-102
Contraindications to travel, 42, 43f
Coronavirus, 86

Cosmetic surgery, 49, 50
Countries
    developing, 76-77, 88
    profiles, 129-130
Creutzfeldt-Jakob Disease, 89
Cruise ship travel
    disabled travelers, 44, 45
    disease prevention, 44
    inspections, 118
    risks, 44

Deaf travelers, 78
Death
    abroad, 45
    automobile fatalities, 45
Deep vein thrombosis, 7, 72-73, 74f, 75
Dengue fever, 17, 18, 75
Dental care
    directory of dentists, 75, 76
    emergencies, 76
    first aid kit, 76
Department of Foreign Affairs and
    Foreign Trade (Canada), 121,
    127
Department of Health (United
    Kingdom), 10, 12, 23, 24f,
    123-124
Department of State (United States),
    18, 21f, 33, 37, 48
Department of Transportation (United
    States), 37, 47, 56
Developing countries, 76-77, 88
Diabetes mellitus, 31, 76-77, 88
Diarrhea, 12, 77-78
Diet, 79
Disabled travelers, 45-47, 103, 113
Disaster preparedness, 52
Disease. *See also* Diarrhea; Malaria;
    SARS
    emerging, 16, 118, 121
    outbreaks, 20, 113, 115-116, 117f,
        118, 120, 129
    risks, 102, 123-124
    statistics, 10, 130
    surveillance, 120-121, 122-123, 129

Dizziness, 42
Dogs, 53-57, 58f
Driving
   directions, 103
   disabled drivers, 45-46
   distance calculators, 103
   fatalities, 45
   international, 36, 37
   with pets, 53-57
   safety, 35, 36, 37, 99, 112
   senior drivers, 37, 38f
   tests, 37, 102
   traffic congestion reports, 104
   winter weather, 36
Drugs
   illegal, 51-52, 121
   prescription, 10-11, 51-52, 121
DVT (deep vein thrombosis), 7, 72-73, 74f, 75

E111 form, 23, 124
Ears, effects of altitude, 78
Ebola virus, 75, 120
Economy class syndrome, 7, 72-73, 74f, 75
Elderly travelers. *See* Senior travelers
Emergency medical treatment, 22, 33, 50
Emerging diseases, 16, 121
Encephalitis, 29, 125
Evacuation, 32, 33, 48, 51
Exercise, 79-80
Expatriate workers, 33

Fear of flying, 80
File transfer protocol (ftp), 1
Fitness, 79-80
Flight delays, 115
Food
   allergies, 66-67, 112
   contamination/poisoning, 81, 82, 115-116, 118
   handling, 81
   safety, 81-82

Foreign and Commonwealth Office (United Kingdom), 10, 17, 96, 109
Forms
   E111, 23, 124
   PHS-731, 25
Frostbite, 72

Gopher, 2

Handicapped travelers, 45-47
Hantavirus, 75
Health certificates, 23, 25, 26, 27, 53, 56
Health examinations, predeparture, 32
Health tourism, 49-50
Hearing-impaired travelers, 78
Heat-related illnesses
   children, 94-95
   cramps, 94
   exhaustion, 93-94
Hemorrhagic fevers, 75
Hepatitis, 82-83, 118
HIV/AIDS
   HIV-positive travelers, 26, 83, 124
   testing requirements, 25, 83
   vaccinations, 26, 28, 124
Hypertext transfer protocol (http), 1
Hypothermia, 72

Immunizations
   certificates, 14, 25, 26, 27
   country-specific, 27, 28, 29, 30f, 130
   HIV/AIDS travelers, 26, 28, 124
   immunocompromised travelers, 28, 83, 124
   pregnant travelers, 27, 29, 92, 123
Immunocompromised travelers, 27, 28, 83, 124
Insects
   bites and stings, 70-71, 95-96
   precautions, 71
Insurance, 32-33, 48
Invisible Web, 6

Jet lag, 7, 8, 84-85, 102-103, 113, 116, 118

Lassa fever, 75
Liver diseases, 82-83, 118
Lung diseases, 85-86, 87f, 88, 127
Lyme disease, 88-89

Mad cow disease, 89
Malaria
   overview, 89-90
   prevention, 90
   risks, 29-30, 90, 130
Maps
   diseases, 102, 125
   driving distances, 103
   national, 37, 103
   traffic congestion reports, 104
   world, 129-130
Medical contraindications, 42, 43f
Medications, 51-52, 121
Meningitis, 12-13
Microorganisms, 115-116, 117f, 123
Mosquitoes, 71, 95-96
Motion sickness, 90-91, 103
Muslim pilgrims, 10, 12, 29, 130

Natural disasters, 52-53
Natural toxins, 123
Neurodegenerative diseases, 89

Organizations, 107-114
Ostomies, 31

Peanut allergies, 66, 67
Pets, 53-57, 58f
PHS-731 form, 25
Plague, 118
Plastic surgery, 49-50

Polar medicine, 71, 109, 124-125
Pregnant travelers
   air travel, 91-93
   developing countries, 88, 92-93
   vaccinations, 27, 29, 92, 123
Pretravel planning, 32
Publications, 115-133

Quarantine
   human, 59
   pets, 54, 59-60

Rage, 65-66
Railroad travel, 39
Respiratory diseases, 85-86, 87f, 88, 127
Road
   closures, 103
   conditions, 36, 103
   maps, 37
   rage, 65, 66
   traffic congestion reports, 104
   traffic safety, 35-37, 99, 112

Safety
   airline, 35-36
   automobile, 35-37, 99, 112
   bus, 39
   train, 39
SARS, 85-86, 87f, 127
Search tools, 4-6
Senior travelers
   automobile driving, 37, 38f
   traveling alone, 12-13, 60, 61f, 62, 121
   traveling with, 60
Severe Acute Respiratory Syndrome (SARS), 85-86, 87f, 127
Shock, anaphylactic, 66-67
Sleep, 84-85

Index

Special-needs travelers
　children, 40
　disabled, 45-47, 113
　HIV/AIDS, 83-84
　immunocompromised, 28, 83
　pets, 53-57, 58f
　pregnant, 27, 29
　seniors, 12-13, 37, 38, 45, 60, 61f, 62, 121
State Department (United States), 56, 63
Statistics
　accidents, 37, 39, 45
　disease, 10, 130
Stings. *See* Bites and stings
Stretching. *See* Exercise
Sun-related ailments
　children, 94-95
　cramps, 94
　first aid, 93
　heat exhaustion, 93-94
　skin cancer, 93
　sunburn, 93
　sunstroke, 93-94
Supplies
　diabetes mellitus, 77
　first aid, 12-13, 21, 31
　ostomy, 31
Surgery, 49-50
Surveillance, disease, 120-121, 122-123, 129

Telnet, 1
Temperatures, 99, 100f, 104
Terrorism, 116, 52
Third world countries, 76-77
Thrombophlebitis, 7, 72-73, 74f, 75
Toothaches. *See* Dental care
Toxins, 115-116, 117f, 123
Traffic
　congestion reports, 104
　safety, 35-37, 99, 112
　warnings, 103
Train travel, 39, 41

Travel
　adventure, 127
　advisories, 25, 105
　agents, 52, 57, 107
　alerts, 12
　checklists, 23, 25-26, 31
　clinics, 8, 10, 16, 17, 20, 48, 105
　contraindications, 42, 43f
　health certificates, 23, 25, 26, 27, 53, 56
　health insurance, 32-33
　medical kits, 12-13, 21, 31
　with pets, 53-57, 58f
　planning, 23-33
　risks, 12, 32
Tropical diseases
　organizations, 107, 129
　publications, 129
Tuberculosis, 85, 88, 127, 129

U. S. Bureau of Consular Affairs, 8, 19f, 20, 37, 52
U. S. Department of State, 18, 21f, 33, 37, 48

Vaccinations
　certificates, 14, 25, 26, 27
　country-specific, 27, 28, 29, 30f, 130
　HIV/AIDS travelers, 26, 28, 124
　immunocompromised travelers, 28, 83, 124
　pregnant travelers, 27, 29, 92, 123
Vertigo, 42

Water purification, 82, 115
Weather
　advisories, 62
　air quality, 101, 103, 105
　national forecasts, 62, 105
　world forecasts, 62, 99, 100f
West Nile virus, 12-13, 95-96

Women traveling alone, 63
World
   country profiles, 129-130
   flags, 129-130
   maps, 129-130
   temperatures, 99, 100f, 104
World Wide Web
   address suffixes, 2t, 3
   evaluating content, 3-4
   general search engines/directories, 4-5

World Wide Web *(continued)*
   invisible, 6
   software, 1, 4
   specialized search engines, 5-6

Yellow fever, 14, 96, 97f, 118

Zoonotic diseases, 120

Order a copy of this book with this form or online at:
http://www.haworthpress.com/store/product.asp?sku=5276

INTERNET GUIDE TO TRAVEL HEALTH

_____ in hardbound at $24.95 (ISBN: 0-7890-1597-8)

_____ in softbound at $14.95 (ISBN: 0-7890-1824-1)

Or order online and use special offer code HEC25 in the shopping cart.

COST OF BOOKS_____

☐ **BILL ME LATER:** (Bill-me option is good on US/Canada/Mexico orders only; not good to jobbers, wholesalers, or subscription agencies.)

☐ Check here if billing address is different from shipping address and attach purchase order and billing address information.

POSTAGE & HANDLING_____
(US: $4.00 for first book & $1.50 for each additional book)
(Outside US: $5.00 for first book & $2.00 for each additional book)

Signature_____

SUBTOTAL_____

☐ **PAYMENT ENCLOSED:** $_____

IN CANADA: ADD 7% GST_____

☐ **PLEASE CHARGE TO MY CREDIT CARD.**

STATE TAX_____
(NY, OH, MN, CA, IIL, N, & SD residents, add appropriate local sales tax)

☐ Visa ☐ MasterCard ☐ AmEx ☐ Discover
☐ Diner's Club ☐ Eurocard ☐ JCB

Account # _____

FINAL TOTAL_____
(If paying in Canadian funds, convert using the current exchange rate, UNESCO coupons welcome)

Exp. Date_____

Signature_____

Prices in US dollars and subject to change without notice.

NAME_____
INSTITUTION_____
ADDRESS_____
CITY_____
STATE/ZIP_____
COUNTRY_____ COUNTY (NY residents only)_____
TEL_____ FAX_____
E-MAIL_____

May we use your e-mail address for confirmations and other types of information? ☐ Yes ☐ No
We appreciate receiving your e-mail address and fax number. Haworth would like to e-mail or fax special discount offers to you, as a preferred customer. **We will never share, rent, or exchange your e-mail address or fax number.** We regard such actions as an invasion of your privacy.

Order From Your Local Bookstore or Directly From
The Haworth Press, Inc.
10 Alice Street, Binghamton, New York 13904-1580 • USA
TELEPHONE: 1-800-HAWORTH (1-800-429-6784) / Outside US/Canada: (607) 722-5857
FAX: 1-800-895-0582 / Outside US/Canada: (607) 771-0012
E-mailto: orders@haworthpress.com

For orders outside US and Canada, you may wish to order through your local sales representative, distributor, or bookseller.
For information, see http://haworthpress.com/distributors

(Discounts are available for individual orders in US and Canada only, not booksellers/distributors.)

PLEASE PHOTOCOPY THIS FORM FOR YOUR PERSONAL USE.

http://www.HaworthPress.com   BOF04